WAKING UP
TO WEED

How Cannabis Can Be Key
to Feeling and Aging Better

**A Guide to New Uses and Benefits
of Marijuana for Your Body, Mind & Life**

Stephanie Byer

For those curious or considering cannabis and for anyone trying to figure out how to navigate this new world of weed, this guide's for you!

Important Note

This book shares my insight and opinions, based upon my experience, secondary research and anecdotal information. It is intended for general informational and educational purposes only. The use and distribution of cannabis are governed by federal and state laws that vary widely; such activities remain illegal in many jurisdictions. Possession, use, cultivation and distribution of cannabis remains federally illegal, regardless of your state law.

This book is not intended to provide legal advice. Educate yourself and seek professional legal guidance as appropriate about current laws and regulations before using or buying cannabis or following any ideas or suggestions in this book. I remind you of your obligation to abide by applicable laws.

It's also not intended to provide medical or health advice, diagnosis or treatment, or to cover all possible uses, benefits, precautions, directions, warnings, guidance or effects. Any statements or claims about possible health benefits and effects have not been evaluated by the FDA or any regulatory organization. Cannabis' effects can vary widely depending on the consumer and consumption. Consult your healthcare professional(s) before using cannabis or following any ideas or suggestions in the book.

I believe the facts and information in this book are accurate as of the date of production; content could include technical inaccuracies or other errors.

Choosing to use cannabis is done at your own risk. I do not assume, and specifically disclaim, any responsibility for any loss, damage, injury or other consequences resulting from anyone's use of cannabis or application of information contained within the book.

—Stephanie Byer

MY SHOUT OUT TO THE LADIES

This book goes out to all the ladies. The moms. The sisters and the aunts. The grandmas. The soul sisters and tribes that help us shine. Thank you.

To the women who've driven, and continue to drive, this cause forward. The old guard hippie generation carried the torch for a generation, sharing their love for the plant and culture surrounding it. The ripple effect of your philosophy of love, acceptance and peace touches everything and will carry forward for generations. Thank you.

To the women who've fought so hard for their children, their loved ones and for themselves. Never enough for themselves. To those who've fought the system. Who've lost loved ones to the system. Who've done whatever it takes to take care of their families. Thank you.

To the women protecting our communities and our rights. Shaping laws and regulations. Driving the ball forward on the path to legalization. Tirelessly fighting the War on Drugs. Defending those unjustly caught up in the War on Drugs and outdated regulations. To those taking the hits along the way. Thank you.

To the women who are shaping and driving a new industry forward, to places we can't even imagine. This industry is in its infancy, this is our weed baby. Let's make sure it grows up to be a healthy, contributing member of society. To those building businesses and brands; creating new opportunities to empower themselves and others. Thank you.

To the plants. The girls. Cannabis is, after all, a female. The mother. The ultimate hippie, and I'm proud to be in her cult. She has given so much to me—I'm grateful and humbled for the opportunity to give her a platform and a chance to be seen for the incredible, powerful little lady she is. Thank you.

And last, but certainly not least, to the woman who raised me. The one who put up with all my shit and loved me through it all. Who exhibited more patience and serenity than anyone could be expected to have without the advantage of weed, particularly in my teen years. Who (and by the way, all of this goes for my dad, too) has supported me fully as I threw my life in the air to pursue a pot-laden path out to Colorado in pursuit of my higher purpose. To my mom. With all my heart and all my love, thank you.

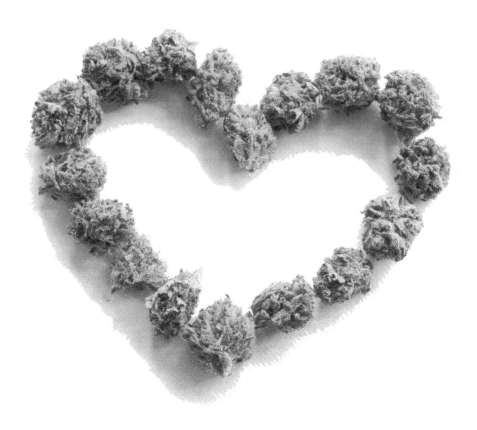

BEFORE
WE
GET
STARTED

After decades of propaganda and stigmatization, marijuana is finally coming out of the closet. As more states legalize and more people open their eyes to its possibilities, there is a vast new world of weed becoming available. But for many, this new world is confusing, overwhelming and perhaps a bit intimidating. Weren't we told marijuana is dangerous and that we should "just say no"? And isn't weed ridiculously strong these days?

If you find yourself with questions about marijuana and wondering where to even start, *Waking Up to Weed* is for you. I've written this book to help you, and anyone considering or questioning cannabis for that matter, understand what's what with regard to weed. It will break down the myths and misperceptions, cover how weed works naturally with our bodies to help a vast range of conditions, help you navigate this new world of weed and show you how it can be safely and guiltlessly incorporated into a healthy, vibrant life. (Spoiler alert: you don't have to get high to get the benefits of marijuana!)

Why *Waking Up to Weed*? Why Now?

Because, despite the fact that support for legalization is at an all-time high, there continues to be misperception and fear around this plant with so much versatility and potential, and it's keeping people from even considering, let alone consuming, cannabis and tapping into its vast range of benefits.

And, because I want to share what I've learned and what I believe about weed. I've developed an understanding of and passion for this plant and what it can do for people and the world around us. I woke up to the full potential and power of pot, and have a deep-rooted desire to help others make their own connection and build their own relationship with cannabis.

Waking Up to Weed synthesizes my knowledge and wisdom gained through many years of secondary research, personal experience and numerous conversations with people inside and outside the marijuana industry. I'm sharing what I've learned to help people become more open-minded, informed and comfortable with the idea that weed is not the addictive, sloth-inducing drug we've been led to believe for as long as most of us have been alive. That it can open up a new world to many people; one with less pain, illness, stress and anxiety and more enjoyment, relaxation, peace and even happiness. And for anyone who does open up to the possibility and want to explore how weed might fit into your life, I also wanted to help you figure out what the heck to do next!

To be clear, I am not a doctor, I'm not making medical claims or promises, nor is this book a medical cannabis resource—there are doctors and experts with far deeper expertise, research and specialized knowledge. This is not a scientific journal, I'm sure there are people who can and will poke holes in points I make in the book. We are in the infancy of research; studies are early, small and scattered. Evidence is scarce. There is debate still to be had and much still to be learned. There is great promise, but little hard proof at this time.

I did not include footnotes, as all facts and stats I include to support my points are readily searchable online and are usually from multiple sources. I will provide resources and further reading suggestions in the appendix, but if there's a fact or a piece of information that you just don't quite buy, I encourage you to go online (you can google just about anything!), do a little research and form your own opinion. That's what I did; I just went the extra mile and put it into a book!

In sharing my point of view, I'm not encouraging you to break the law and put anyone at risk. I do believe weed should be legalized, but until that happens, marijuana is still illegal on a federal level, and not yet legally available in every state. I am not a lawyer nor do I have any expertise in the law, our rights, regulations, compliance or any other area of practice that requires training and licensing.

But, I have done my homework and present my perspective and position on pot. You may disagree, disbelieve or discount some of the assertions I make or the information I present—I encourage you to dig in and form your own perspective. Every data point or fact in here was pulled from publicly available content. If you don't trust my synthesis or want more back-up, there's plenty out there. If you don't agree with my perspective, that's okay too. I don't expect everyone to agree with me or believe every point I make. For some, I won't be able to defend my points to their satisfaction. Others may have a personal experience that overshadows everything else. It's all good, I'm passionate about this plant, but I'm not militant or strident that I'm right and anyone who disagrees is wrong; or that everyone has to get on board the train to Weedtown.

I don't expect everyone to share my passion or embrace weed as a way of life. I am not promoting weed as a panacea for everything; it is not for every person and it is not a miracle cure. But I do want everyone to open their eyes to what's possible and make a conscious choice about what relationship, if any, to have with cannabis.

What I do want with all my heart is for you to walk away from this book with at least one piece of information that surprises you, teaches you something new and shifts your perspective, even if it's just a tiny bit. When you finish the book, if you don't walk away having learned something new, I will have failed. And if I can give you more than a new piece of information or insight and actually help in some way, I will be deeply grateful. I hope the book will open your eyes and your mind, and will surprise and entertain you along the way. Perhaps it will spark a conversation and open up new possibilities.

Oh, and on a final note:

Waking Up to Weed is intended to be a practical, information-rich guide to marijuana, the many ways it can help so many people and the many ways it can be consumed and enjoyed. I've crammed a lot in here—it is comprehensive and covers pretty much everything about weed on some level. I don't expect all of it will be relevant or interesting to you. It's okay. Skip around. Dive into questions or topics of interest. Skim. Go back for a refresh. You don't have to read this from cover to cover. Much as you will choose your own path when it comes to pot, you can choose your own path through this book. There's no one way to consume it. Just like weed!

WEED, IT'S NOT JUST FOR STONERS ANYMORE

Hi there, or rather, *high there!*

If you're reading this, I'm going to assume you are new to the world of weed (or cannabis, as we call it today), or at least are returning to it after some time away. Welcome (back)! Don't be afraid. It's a far different world than you've been led to believe. And, nothing like the experience you had back in college.

For anyone over the age of 40, marijuana has been framed as the gateway to all sorts of evil sins. Addiction. Drug abuse. Sloth. Stupidity. Crime. Paranoid delusions. Political dissent.

What if I told you that just about everything you've been told, and likely, everything you believe, about marijuana is wrong?

That it's not addictive or dangerous, it won't do harm to your body or brain, and you cannot overdose. (You can, however, have a bad experience by eating too much and end up feeling really, really uncomfortable. Maureen Dowd of the *New York Times* is now the cautionary tale told throughout the land to "go low and slow." She recklessly ate an entire 100 mg edible (despite being cautioned otherwise) and paid the price. But, it's easily avoidable, I'll tell you how!)

That its status as a Schedule 1 drug by our federal government is in direct conflict with government-funded research and is a direct result of demonization by politicians with personal prejudices who completely ignored the evidence and recommendations from their own commissions.

That it is, for many, an exit ramp from addiction, opioids, pain and an ever-increasing range of afflictions (more to come on its health benefits in a bit). That there hasn't been one marijuana-related overdose or death. (Opioid overdoses kill 91 Americans each day.) That it stops seizures and spasms, can be as effective as opioids for pain management, kills cancer cells and attacks the plaque that causes Alzheimer's. And that's just the tip of the iceberg.

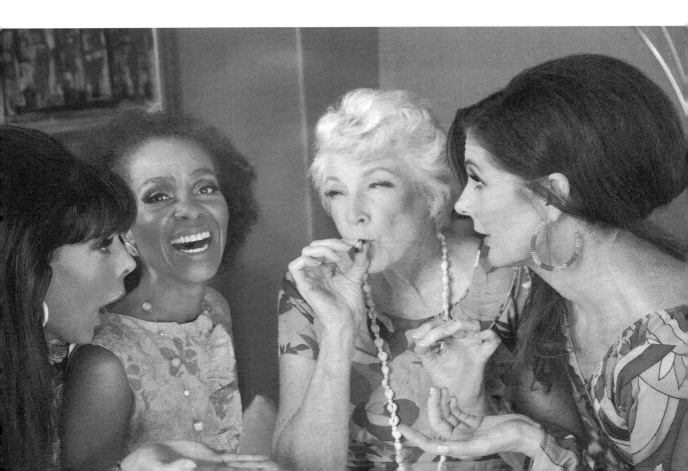

If anything, marijuana is a gateway to enhanced experiences, better health and greater happiness.

I've had hundreds of conversations with people living outside the "weed bubble," and I continue to be surprised at how little knowledge has made it into the mainstream. How much misperception and misinformation continues, blocking people from finding healing and relief. How few people understand their choices when it comes to consumption and that they have options which don't involve getting high or firing up a joint. And how much opportunity there is to help bring light to this misrepresented and maligned plant.

Even if you're not surprised, there's a good chance you're overwhelmed and apprehensive about this new world of weed. Even if you know someone who sparks up or medicates, there's a good chance you have little idea of what's available, how to navigate your choices, what questions to ask and where to even start. And even if you've taken a hit or tried an edible, there's far more to know about cannabis.

Oh yeah, there's also a good chance someone you know is on board with the benefits of weed, even if they're not out of the closet. Cannabis is now legal in more than half the United States (despite remaining illegal federally). Public support is at an all-time high: a recent Gallup poll showed 64% of Americans think it should be legal. When it comes to medical marijuana, support skyrockets to nearly 90%.

Middle-aged Americans are now more likely to toke up than their teenaged kids. The percentage of American adults who say they consume marijuana has nearly doubled in just three years, with some of the biggest growth coming from women and Baby Boomers. In fact, the 55+ crowd is the fastest growing demographic of pot users in the country. Retirees are swapping bridge for a sesh (smoke session…read on, I'll give you the lingo!). Suburban soccer moms are unwinding with weed instead of wine. And millions are dropping their opioids and other medications for weed.

> **The stoner stereotype is going up in smoke. If you think people who partake are lazy, unsuccessful and apathetic, think again.**

I, for instance, am an accomplished, successful professional with social and business skills who smokes weed. I've enjoyed it socially for the majority of my adult life. I've benefited from it as I took on breast cancer, opioid addiction and chronic pain. I turned my life upside down and left a comfortable life and job in New York City to dive head first into the cannabis industry. I wake up each day in gratitude, live in the present and am more mindful with cannabis as part of my life.

I'm not an exception. A recent study showed those who do consume cannabis are among the most satisfied and successful among us. Like me, my fellow potheads are more content with life and are accomplished professionally and personally. Oh, we're thinner, more active, and have better sex lives too.

Surprise!

So, if you're curious about cannabis and want to figure out if it might be for you, someone you care about or even your pet… read on. I'll break down the "whats" and "hows" of weed, the misperceptions and myths and the many ways in which it can bring benefits to multitudes. I'll give you guidance on how to get started and navigate an ever-expanding range of products and choices. And you'll see how weed can be incorporated into a healthy, vibrant lifestyle that is far from Doritos and video games.

Marijuana isn't for everyone. I'm not trying to lure you into a cult of cannabis. But I do want you to see its potential, and to help you overcome the stigma and misperceptions that might be keeping you or someone you love from healing or finding relief. And if nothing else, I want you to be able to stay current as marijuana moves into the mainstream and onto Main Street. At the very least, you should know how to respond if your neighbor asks you over for a sesh!

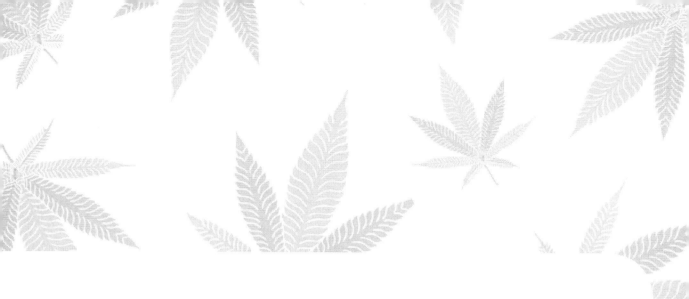

CLOSING QUESTION

If weed isn't really bad, why does everyone think it is?

Well, first of all, not everyone does think it's bad. People with all levels of experience and expertise are coming to realize that, in reality, cannabis provides significant therapeutic potential and benefits; with none of the risk and bad behavior we've been imprinted to associate with weed. The vast majority of Americans support medical marijuana in some form, and a growing majority—more than 60%—support legalization. But the stigma is sticky. Some people are still judge-y, though likely fewer than you think. That said, we've been programmed to be hysterical and paranoid, so it's going to take time for people to lose the (perceived) stigma and misperception. It starts with knowledge, so keep reading to learn more about pot and its possibilities.

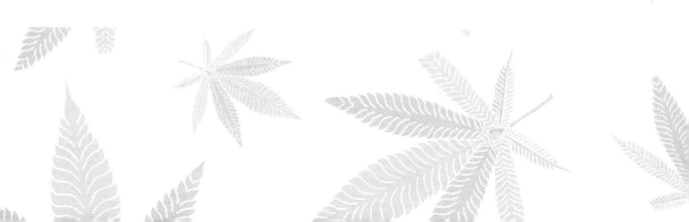

(RE)INTRODUCING YOURSELF TO WEED: IT'S NOTHING LIKE YOU FEAR

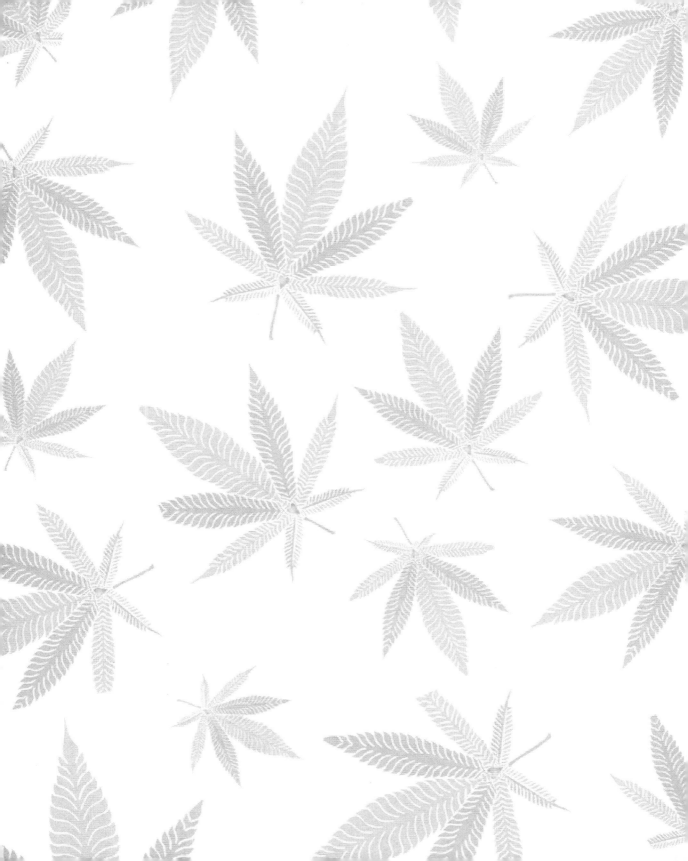

1 | YOU DON'T KNOW WHAT YOU DON'T KNOW

I've smoked weed since college. My ex-husband used to grow fantastic bud in our basement. Amongst my friends and colleagues, I was the "pothead." I had a favorite strain (Sour Diesel). I thought I was an expert. Then I decided to put my professional sights on the cannabis industry and moved to Colorado to learn the consumer market from the inside out.

I had no idea what I didn't know.

My knowledge, experience and vocabulary have expanded exponentially. I've tried hundreds of new products, ways to consume and strains (Sour Diesel remains my favorite). Talked to hundreds of budtenders (exactly as it sounds, the ones who serve you at a dispensary), product manufacturers, entrepreneurs, growers and other cannabis experts. Spent hundreds of hours reading and absorbing new information as it emerges from the various reaches of the interweb.

There is always something new to learn. Always.

Federally funded research on the benefits of cannabis is prohibitive and limited, thanks to its continued status as a Schedule 1 drug, alongside heroin, LSD and ecstasy. (Sidenote: both LSD and MDMA, the street name for ecstasy, are undergoing federally funded studies for treatment of depression and PTSD. In fact, the FDA just proclaimed MDMA to be a "breakthrough drug" for treating PTSD and is fast tracking the drug to clinical trials. You might be surprised about these drugs, too. But that's for another book!)

SIDE EFFECTS YOU ACTUALLY WANT

The DEA, which continues to go to the mat defending marijuana's Schedule 1 status, publishes a resource guide: Drugs of Abuse. It acknowledges that no deaths from marijuana have ever been reported. The side effects? "Merriment," "happiness," "enhanced sensory perception," "increased appreciation of music, art and touch," and "heightened imagination." I ask you: What's the problem with these side effects?

Despite these constraints, more and more research is emerging to back up what various cultures have known for literally ages: cannabis is a plant with remarkable abilities to heal, to connect people to their spirituality and to each other, to enhance experiences and lives. It's also good for the planet, so there's that.

So, here we are, at the threshold of a massive shift in awareness and acceptance of marijuana. Our collective understanding of this surprising plant has been muddled by politics and personal morality; what we think we know isn't the real story.

Let's start with a brief history lesson on marijuana and how it became the victim of a propaganda campaign that began back in the '30s and continued well into the '80s. The impact has been far-reaching and damaging, fueling a prison industry disproportionate with young, black men and ruining countless lives. All for a natural substance far less dangerous than alcohol.

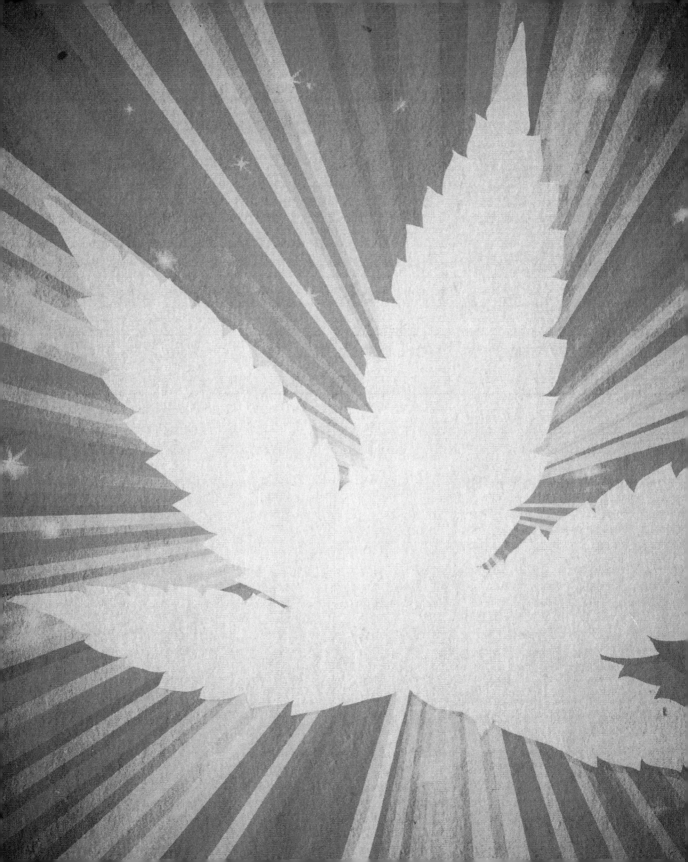

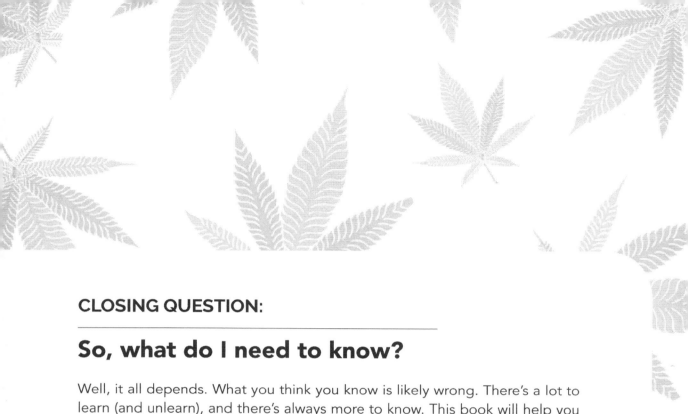

CLOSING QUESTION:

So, what do I need to know?

Well, it all depends. What you think you know is likely wrong. There's a lot to learn (and unlearn), and there's always more to know. This book will help you know what you need to know— what you get from it will be driven by what you already know, what you want to know and where you want to go with all this newfound knowledge! To start, the fundamental lesson goes as follows: marijuana isn't bad or dangerous, and in fact is pretty much the polar opposite.

2 | HUMANITY'S HISTORY WITH THE HERB

Across the globe and over the course of history, people have used cannabis medicinally, religiously, recreationally and spiritually. Earliest evidence of cannabis shows up around 12,000 years ago. Multiple archeological digs have uncovered cannabis seeds and cultivation evidence. The spread of medicinal cannabis first started in China, then traveled throughout Asia into the Middle East and Africa. Texts from ancient India acknowledge its psychoactive properties, and doctors used it for ailments from pain to insomnia, headaches to gastrointestinal disorders. Use was widespread and accepted as treatment for pain and a vast range of conditions. Even Queen Victoria supposedly used cannabis tea to help her relieve her monthly cramps.

So, it's both renewable and can be incorporated into thousands of products: anywhere from 25,000 to 50,000 products, impressive numbers on either end of the range! It can't get you high. And it helps make our planet a better place. Hemp being classified as a Schedule 1 drug simply makes no sense. Cannabis has been used as medicine for thousands of years. Way back in ancient times, it was recognized as one of 50 'fundamental herbs' by Chinese medicine and prescribed for a wide range of ailments and conditions. Westerners were a little later to the game, catching on to the concept in the 1800s when an Irish doctor with the British East India Company, William O'Shaughnessy, learned of its use while in India and brought this knowledge to his colleagues and peers back home. Cannabis was included in the 1850 edition of the medical reference book *United States Pharmacopeia*, and remained part of it until 1942.

HEMP: A VERSATILE AND INCREDIBLE INDUSTRIAL PRODUCT CAUGHT UP BY CLASSIFICATION

Keep in mind: hemp doesn't get you high. There's nothing about it that can be abused. It's no different than any other agricultural crop. And yet, it is considered cannabis by the letter of the law.

Hemp was—and can be—used for many things: clothes, cars, plastics, building materials, rope, paper, linens, food, medicine and more. Seeds and flowers are used in health foods, organic body care, and other nutraceuticals. Fibers and stalks are used in hemp clothing, construction materials (hempcrete is really a thing), paper, biofuel, plastic composites and more. Henry Ford's first Model-T was built to run on hemp gasoline and the car itself was constructed from hemp!

As it grows, hemp takes in carbon dioxide, detoxifies the soil and prevents soil erosion. It leaves valuable nutrients behind after harvest. And, it requires much less water to grow—and no pesticides—so it is far more environmentally friendly than traditional crops.

For much of human history, cannabis has been used not only for its medicinal, spiritual and intoxicating properties, but also for the fiber and food from the stalks of the plant. Hemp, you may be surprised to hear, is cannabis, just without THC and its psychoactive properties. Ancient cultures used hemp as a common agricultural crop—harvested for its high-protein seeds, oil and fiber used for rope and clothes. At one point, 90% of all ships' sails and rope were made from hemp. In fact, the word 'canvas' comes from the root word 'cannabis.'

Fast forward to colonists settling America; they brought cannabis with them in the form of hemp. Even the sails of the Mayflower were woven with hemp fiber. American colonies were actually required by law to grow hemp because of its vital importance to shipping and industry. Perhaps you've heard that George Washington and many of the Founding

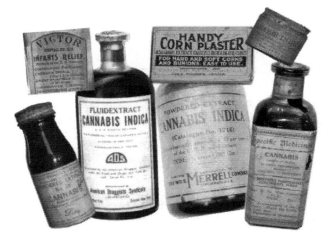

Fathers grew hemp. The Declaration of Independence was written on paper made from hemp fiber. The first flag of the United States, sewn by Betsy Ross, was made of hemp. All true! For a time after the Revolutionary War, farmers could even pay their taxes in hemp.

Marijuana, hemp's cousin that will get you high, didn't come onto the scene until the early 1900s, when the flood of immigrants from the Mexican Revolution poured into the United States. They brought their culture, customs and language over the border, including "marihuana" and its use for pleasure and relaxation. While cannabis was present in almost all tinctures and medicines at the time, "marihuana" was new and foreign.

Public fears, whipped up by a media frenzy, came to rest on this new immigrant population and the demonization of marijuana began. A conscious effort to connect cannabis to foreigners and criminals by calling it "marihuana" and campaigning against its evils was fabricated, insidious and enduring. It took the plant from an accepted medicine and valuable agricultural crop to something to be feared, and ultimately swept it all away in the trail of prohibition and the War on Drugs.

Let's take a look at how this happened. You'll be surprised at how misled you've been.

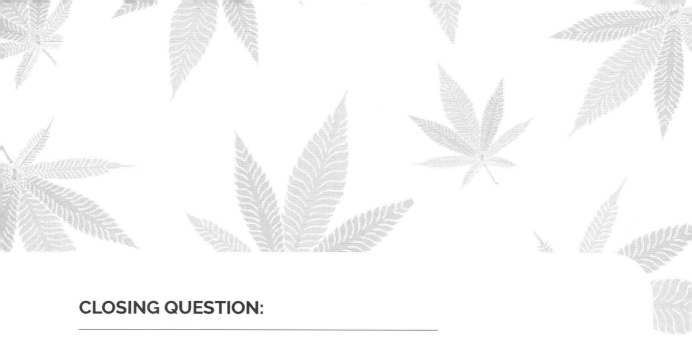

CLOSING QUESTION:

Wait, what? Hemp is cannabis?

Technically hemp is considered cannabis, which has been safely used by humans for thousands of years. Although it can't get you high and has only industrial application, our government still considers it a Schedule 1 drug with a high potential for abuse, no medicinal value and no safe way to consume it. In reality, hemp is an agricultural, industrial crop that can help sustain our planet; contribute value across multiple dimensions; help people and communities; and fuel thousands of products that benefit thousands of people and pets.

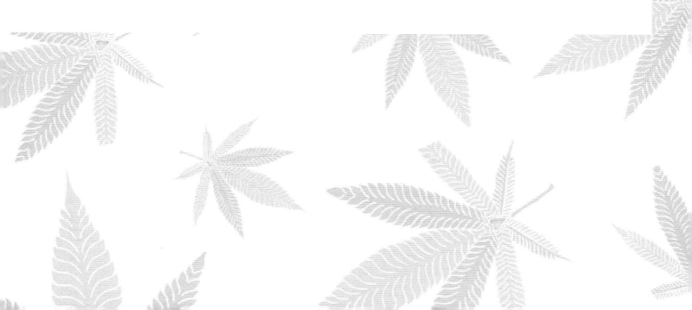

3 | THE MADNESS OF REEFER MADNESS

Let me introduce you to some of the most detested players in the history of marijuana pro-hibition, people who vilified everything about the plant and the people who used it, and who created long-lasting damage to people and society that persists to this day.

It all started in the 30s with Harry Anslinger, head of the newly formed Federal Bureau of Narcotics. Left without job security after Prohibition was repealed, he set his sights on marijuana. Prior to the end of alcohol prohibition, Anslinger had claimed that cannabis was not a problem, did not harm people, and "there is no more absurd fallacy" than the idea it makes people violent. But, as the original architect of the War on Drugs and national Prohibition, he recognized the need to feed the engine, so to speak. Marijuana, with its core user base of Mexican immigrants and African-Americans, was an easy and fruitful target.

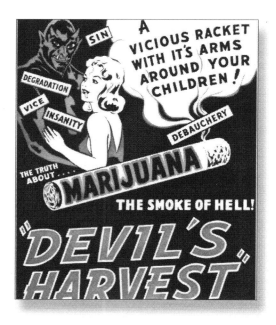

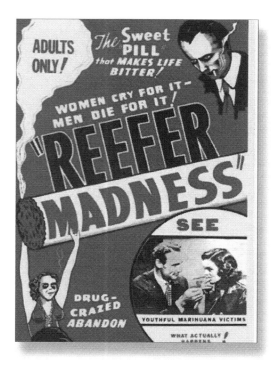

He rested his case on the assertion that marijuana caused insanity and pushed people to criminal behavior. He claimed that black people and Latinos were the primary users of marijuana, and it made them forget their place in the fabric of American society. Tapping into cultural anxieties of racism and xenophobia having nothing to do with the drug, he claimed that it promoted interracial mixing and relationships. The word "marijuana" itself was part of this approach. What was commonly known as cannabis until the early 1900s was now dubbed marihuana, a Spanish word more likely to be associated with Mexican, in order to whip up a racism-based fear frenzy.

He may not have actually believed his propaganda, but as he worked to get Congress to bring marijuana under federal control, he fed the fear and added fuel to the fire by giving lurid stories to the press as a way of making a case for federal intervention. His propaganda gave rise to melodramatic exploitation films *Reefer Madness* and *Assassin of Youth* and a slew of stories in the mass media. In particular, he found an ally in William Randolph Hearst, newspaper magnate and fellow hater of Mexican immigrants.

Hearst published tales of marijuana-crazed Mexicans going on murderous rampages, headlines which sold lots of papers. But it wasn't just the headlines Hearst was after. As they say, follow the money. In this case, the money trail leads to the forest.

Newspapers are made out of wood pulp, an industry in which—shocker—Hearst had heavily invested. Hemp, which had not been cost effective to produce, suddenly became a viable option with new technology. It was now possible to make paper cheaper, in less time and with less environmental impact than logging. Hearst's big investment was in big jeopardy. Keeping hemp illegal was of critical importance to Hearst.

With the growing hysteria from what might be the world's most effective and nefarious branding campaign, Anslinger was able help introduce and pass the Marijuana Tax Act of 1937, drafted by Anslinger and which effectively made possession, transfer or sale of cannabis illegal. He did this despite objections from the American Medical Association and contacting 30 scientists for scientific evidence; 29 told him cannabis was not a dangerous drug.

> " Marijuana is taken by musicians.
> And I'm not speaking about good musicians,
> but the jazz type. "

HARRY J. ANSLINGER
Federal Bureau of Narcotics, 1948

In response to the Marijuana Tax Act, then-Mayor of New York Fiorello LaGuardia commissioned a report to confirm his suspicions: that marijuana did not impact a person's sensibilities or ability to make good decisions and that it likely was not as dangerous as Anslinger and his buddies were making it out to be with their "Reefer Madness" campaign. The LaGuardia Committee reports systematically contradicted claims that smoking marijuana results in insanity, deteriorates physical and mental health, assists in criminal behavior and juvenile delinquency, is addictive and is a "gateway" drug to more dangerous drugs.

Anslinger was infuriated. He condemned the report, calling it unscientific. He denounced LaGuardia, the New York Academy of Medicine and the doctors who had worked for more than five years on the research. He continued his war against weed, remaining in power for 32 years.

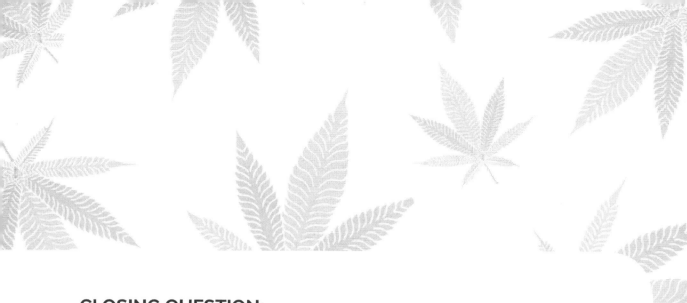

CLOSING QUESTION:

You mean politics and prejudice are behind the pot stigma?

Yup. All propaganda fabricated and promoted by a bureaucrat seeking a reason for professional existence. There was no proof for any claims of reefer rampages. The media fueled a public frenzy that had nothing and yet everything to do with weed. There is no basis whatsoever for our belief system that marijuana is a gateway to shocking and immoral behavior. Until it was rebranded as marijuana and saddled with its false and fear-based associations, cannabis was medicine, a non-issue until a desperate politician made it one.

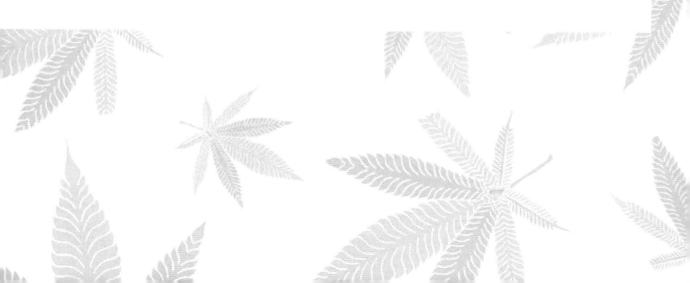

4 | THE WAR ON DRUGS THAT WAS NEVER WON

It was 1971 when President Richard Nixon declared his infamous (and incalculably damaging) War on Drugs. We know now from recordings and former staff that this war was contrived by a paranoid, prejudiced prevaricator, with sights set on two enemies: hippies and blacks. Nixon created the War on Drugs to bully his political enemies and minorities, giving him the tools to essentially criminalize being anti-war or black. These White House tapes reveal that Nixon's opinions about marijuana were based on his personal prejudices rather than the evidence. He believed the marijuana legalization movement to be a Jewish conspiracy, and that it fueled political dissent. By getting the public to associate the hippies with marijuana and blacks with heroin, and then criminalizing both heavily, he could disrupt those communities and vilify them night after night on the evening news.

Yet again, the foundation for the war on marijuana was prejudice, culture war and misinformation.

The next big battle in the war came in 1970, when Congress passed the Controlled Substances Act. It temporarily classified marijuana as a Schedule 1 drug, a designation reserved for intoxicants with the highest potential for abuse and no accepted medical use. But Congress acknowledged that it did not know enough about marijuana to permanently relegate it to Schedule I, and so they created a presidential commission to review the research and recommend a long-term strategy.

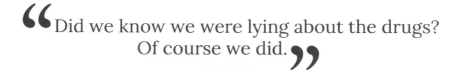

"Did we know we were lying about the drugs? Of course we did. "

JOHN ERLICHMAN

White House Domestic Affairs Advisor, 1969—1973

President Nixon, fueled by his personal vendetta against pot, convened the Shafer Commission to engineer scientific support for cannabis's Schedule I placement. Led by former Republican Governor of Pennsylvania and "law and order" prosecutor, Raymond Shafer, the Commission was loaded with drug warriors, congressmen, the dean of a law school, the head of a mental health hospital, scientists and law enforcement officials. The Shafer Commission took its job seriously. They launched 50 research projects, polled the public and members of the criminal justice community and took thousands of pages of testimony. Their work is still the most comprehensive review of marijuana ever conducted by the federal government.

After two years of study, the report, "Marihuana: A Signal of Misunderstanding," was a surprise to everyone. It called for the end of prohibition. After a deep dive into all the evidence, these drug warriors were forced to come to a different conclusion than they had expected. Rather than being an addictive, damaging drug, marijuana did not lead to harder drug use or cause damage to mind or body. Rather than harshly condemning marijuana, they started talking about legalization.

> **"Considering the range of social concerns in contemporary America, marihuana does not, in our considered judgment, rank very high. We would deemphasize marihuana as a problem. Marihuana's relative potential for harm to the vast majority of individual users and its actual impact on society does not justify a social policy designed to seek out and firmly punish those who use it."**

Nixon did not get what he wanted. He flat-out rejected and shelved his own commission's call to decriminalize marijuana. Based on his zealous personal preferences, he overruled the commission's research and doomed marijuana to its current illegal status.

In 1982, Nancy Reagan uttered the words "Just say no" and thus was born the rallying cry for a generation of adolescent drug-prevention programs. The most publicized program, D.A.R.E., was the one I, and just about every youth behind me, grew up on. Drug Abuse Resistance Education, better known by its acronym, was created in 1983 by the Los Angeles Police Department and used by roughly 80% of school districts.

Despite being a popular and politically touted program, it is acknowledged by most to be an abject failure. Every study since 1992 on the effectiveness of D.A.R.E., including a major 10-year investigation by the American Psychological Association, has consistently shown that it is ineffective in reducing the use of alcohol and drugs and in fact is even counterproductive—leading to higher drug use and therefore worse than doing nothing. The U.S. Surgeon General categorized it as an "ineffective program" and D.A.R.E. lost federal funding in 1998. Yet, the program hangs on somehow.

Across the board, the War on Drugs has been deemed a failure at every level; headlines affirm "the War on Drugs is lost." From the *New York Times* to the *National Review*, the consensus is this drug war was not, in fact, for the nation's own good. Billions of dollars are thrown away each year in the enforcement of pointless laws. Criminalization has been destructive beyond repair. The United States has the highest incarceration rate in the world, with disproportionately high rates for men of color.

According to an analysis by the Washington Post, in 2016 someone in the U.S. was arrested every 48 seconds for marijuana possession. And according to the ACLU, between 2001 and 2010, more than 50% of all arrests were for marijuana—nearly 90% of those arrests were for simple possession. Not trafficking, distribution or other hardcore crimes. Not drug kingpins. In 2011, there were more arrests for marijuana possession than for all violent crimes put together.

A couple of joints and people have seen extensive jail time (15 years in Louisiana!). Black and brown people are getting arrested at rates nearly four times higher than whites (despite using pot at about the same rate). Countless lives are ruined by outrageously long jail sentences, arrest records that affect jobs, loans, housing and benefits. Police departments waste time and money chasing down a drug that's legal in, and supported by, more than half the United States. In 2011, around 750,000 people were arrested for marijuana-related crimes—that's one arrest every 42 seconds.

The social costs of the marijuana laws are vast. There were 658,000 arrests for marijuana possession in 2012, according to F.B.I. figures, compared with 256,000 for cocaine, heroin and their derivatives. Even worse, the result is racist, falling disproportionately on young black men, ruining their lives and creating new generations of career criminals.

Each year, enforcing laws on possession costs more than $3.6 billion. A report focused on the budgetary impact of prohibition estimated that legalizing drugs would save roughly $41.3 billion per year in government expenditure on enforcement of prohibition. Marijuana legalization would reduce the need for prosecutorial, judicial, correctional and police resource spending by roughly $10 billion per year.

A SPOTLIGHT ON
DRUG SCHEDULING

Schedule I: No currently accepted medical use and a high potential for abuse. Some examples: heroin, LSD, marijuana, ecstasy, methaqualone, and peyote.

Schedule II: A high potential for abuse, potentially leading to severe psychological or physical dependence. These drugs are also considered dangerous. Some examples: Vicodin, cocaine, methamphetamine, methadone, Dilaudid, Demerol, OxyContin, fentanyl, Dexedrine, Adderall and Ritalin.

Schedule III: Moderate to low potential for physical and psychological dependence. Some examples: Tylenol with codeine, ketamine, anabolic steroids and testosterone.

Schedule IV: Low potential for abuse and low risk of dependence. Some examples: Xanax, Soma, Darvon, Darvocet, Valium, Ativan, Talwin, Ambien and Tramadol.

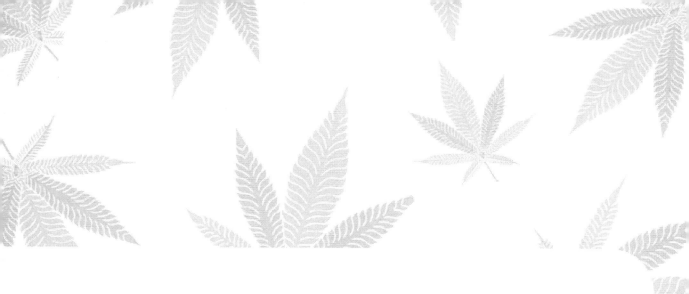

CLOSING QUESTION:

Is waging a war on drugs worth it?

Nope. Nixon's War on Drugs wasn't against drugs, it was against hippies and blacks. There was never a problem, and no need for a war. By giving marijuana Schedule 1 status (in direct conflict with an independent commission's recommendation), Nixon gave permission for authorities to use weed as an excuse to arrest minorities for relatively minor offenses. The War on Drugs costs billions of dollars per year, ruins countless lives and has been called an abject failure across the board. So, no. Not worth it at all.

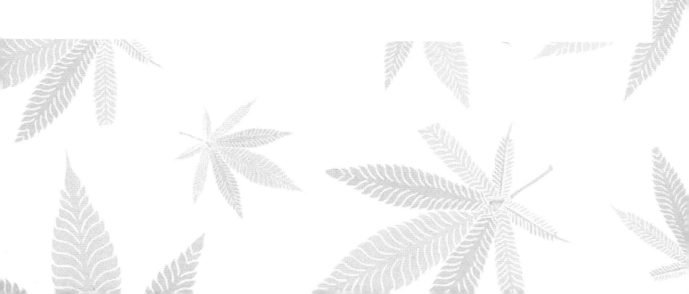

5 | THE WAR WAGES ON

We may not have Anslinger or Nixon leading the charge and fabricating propaganda and political campaigns, and we may have far greater access to marijuana today; but the impact remains and constrains progress, continuing to amass enormous financial and social costs. The misinformation and continued assertions of marijuana's evils despite increasing evidence to the contrary continues. Denials and inconsistencies, flat-out refusals to acknowledge facts, dissemination of blatantly erroneous information about cannabis and ignoring authoritative academic work continue to this day.

The DEA considers marijuana to be as dangerous as heroin, and less so than cocaine and deadly painkillers like fentanyl...yet the U.S. Government holds multiple patents on cannabis, including #6630507 filed nearly 20 years ago, which proves not only its medical benefit but also that it is nontoxic and therefore nonlethal. The hypocrisy runs deep and far, my friends.

U.S PATENT #6630507

Cannabinoids have been found to have antioxidant properties for the treatment and prevention of a wide variety of inflammatory and autoimmune diseases. Cannabinoids are found to be neuroprotectants following stroke and trauma or in the treatment of neurodegenerative diseases, such as Alzheimer's disease, Parkinson's disease and dementia.

As I write this book, a federal lawsuit was filed against the U.S. Government, challenging the constitutionality of classifying cannabis as a Schedule 1 drug. It claims that the federal government does not, and could not possibly, believe (and never has believed) that cannabis meets the definition of a Schedule 1 drug: high potential for abuse, no medical use in treatment and no ability to be used or tested safely, even under medical supervision. And, indeed, the government has admitted repeatedly in writing and through national policy that cannabis does in fact have medical uses and can be used and tested safely under medical supervision. The federal government has exploited cannabis economically for more than a decade by securing a medical cannabis patent and entering into license agreements with medical licensees. We'll see where it shakes out, but it's one more credible example of the hypocrisy behind continued prohibition.

A vast gap remains between antiquated federal enforcement policies and the clear consensus of science that marijuana is far less harmful to human health than other banned drugs, and is less dangerous than the highly addictive but perfectly legal substances known as alcohol and tobacco. Marijuana cannot lead to a fatal overdose. It's not a gateway drug. It's not physically addictive. The myths have been disproven. Yet, they perpetuate.

Cannabis is the world's most consumed, most widely grown and most confiscated drug. Despite its worldwide popularity, not one single person has died from cannabis use. Not in 2015. Not ever. But in 2015, there were nearly 200,000 drug-related deaths, which the United Nations Office on Drugs and Crime (UNODC) believes "is most likely an underestimate." A quarter of all drug-related deaths that year occurred in North America.

"Mostly driven by opioids, overdose deaths more than tripled in the period 1999–2015 and increased by 11.4% in the past year alone, to reach the highest level ever recorded. Of the 52,000 total drug-related deaths reported for the United States, those related to opioids accounted for more than 60%." When broken down by individual drugs, opioids had a significantly higher impact on healthy living, and cannabis had the least harmful impact. We are in the midst of a national crisis, officially recognized and declared so by our government in October 2017.

So, not a single death. Alcohol, on the other hand, kills 88,000 people a year. Tobacco, perfectly legal despite its proven damaging health effects, kills 480,000 people a year.

Beyond death, alcohol can leave a trail of destruction behind it. Alcohol damages the brain. Cannabis does not. In fact, cannabis protects the brain. More on that in a bit.

Drunk driving, domestic violence, addiction and other issues make alcohol far more damaging to society than marijuana. An independent study in Britain compared 20 drugs in 2010 for the harms they caused to individual users and to society as a whole through crime, family breakdown, absenteeism, and other social ills. Adding up all the damage, the panel estimated that alcohol was the most harmful drug, followed by heroin and crack cocaine.

As cliche as it sounds, people who blaze up tend to be chill and stay out of trouble.

ALCOHOL VS. WEED
Open your eyes to a safer, healthier alternative

The true gateway drug	The proven exit drug
Addictive	No physical addiction
Lethal dose = 10 drinks	Lethal dose = none (40,000 joints)
Millions of deaths/year	Zero deaths EVER
Causes cancer	Cures cancer
Destroys and damages cells	Protects, grows and repairs cells
Effects: hangover, nausea, poor decision making, aggression, blackout, depression	Effects: relaxation, relief, rest, peacefulness, ease, happiness, inspiration, laughter
Increases waistlines and blood pressure	May reduce BMI, blood pressure and blood sugar
Fosters violent crime, domestic violence and sexual assault	Fosters peace and love, mindfulness and a hot sex life
Legal	Illegal

Today is a Moving Target

Despite its widespread use and acceptance by an ever-increasing majority of Americans for both medical and recreational use, marijuana remains federally illegal even though three quarters of the United States have legalized some form of it. Thirty states have now legalized medical marijuana; as of January 2018, recreational use is legal in Alaska, California, Colorado, Maine, Massachusetts, Nevada, Oregon and Washington state (and if you're in Washington D.C., you can't buy it, but you can grow it). In its first month of coming online, Nevada already faced a weed crisis; demand so outstripped supply that it created a shortage.

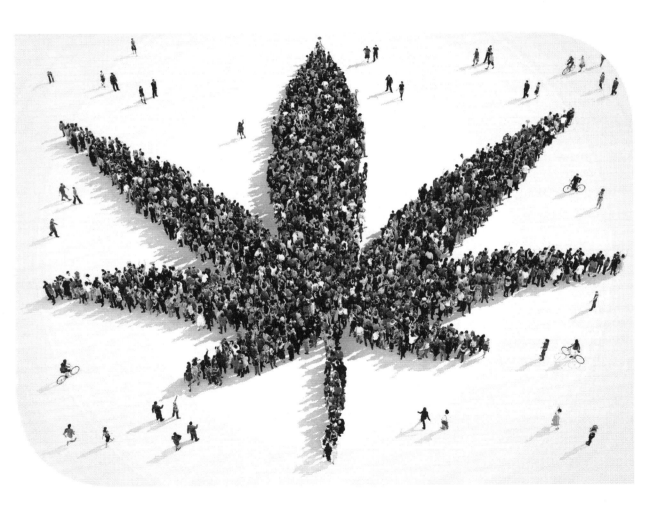

The implications of federal prohibition are far-reaching. Banking isn't available to businesses or individuals associated with the industry. Massive amounts of cash have to be moved, used to pay employees, business expenses and taxes, among many other things. Legit business owners show up to pay taxes at federal buildings with sackfuls of cash. It's dangerous and perpetuates a stereotype of back-alley drug dealing. Businesses that provide ancillary products and services like storage bags and don't even "touch the plant" can't get credit card processing because of their association with cannabis. Dispensary owners who are operating fully within the confines of the law are getting raided (by the government, not by bandits) and facing massive asset forfeiture.

> **"**We have been terribly and systematically misled for nearly 70 years in the United States, and I apologize for my own role in that.**"**

DR. SANJAY GUPTA
American Neurosurgeon and Medical Reporter

Without federal oversight, regulations are state-by-state, and therefore inconsistent. Many states are just beginning to check for unapproved pesticides in cannabis products, while some have no testing program at all. The EPA won't regulate cannabis crops, leaving consumers unprotected. (Big Ag, specifically Scott's Miracle-Gro, has already tried to register pesticides for growing pot.)

Interstate travel and transport of cannabis is illegal, creating operational and distribution challenges for cannabis businesses. States are benefiting from tax revenue—Colorado has pulled in over $500 million in tax revenue since retail sales began in 2014. That revenue has gone mostly to improve schools, with additional revenue funneled to help the homeless, fund drug treatment and prevention programs and finance law enforcement. Oh yeah, drunk driving is down too.

Oh, and for anyone concerned asking "What about our youth?" Well, teen use in Colorado actually went down by 12% after weed became legal. Surprise! That said, legalization may be changing attitudes in a way that encourages adolescent use, and so having a well-regulated system with protections for our youth is critical as more states come online.

On the opposite end of the age spectrum, according to a report in *Health Affairs*, states with medical marijuana saw Medicare prescriptions for drugs used to treat chronic pain, anxiety or depression drop after legalization. Ranges vary, from a 42% reduction in prescriptions to treat nausea to a 13% decline in antidepressant drugs. Prescriptions for drugs like opioid painkillers and antidepressants—and associated Medicare spending on those drugs—fell in states where marijuana could feasibly be used as a replacement (note that prescriptions didn't drop for medicines such as blood-thinners, for which marijuana isn't an alternative). Medical marijuana could have saved Medicare about $165 million in 2013; if it were available nationwide, Medicare Part D spending would have declined in the same year by about $470 million. If all states had legalized medical marijuana in 2014, Medicaid could have saved $1 billion in spending on prescriptions.

Big Pharma is not happy. As the saying goes, the pharmaceutical industry doesn't create cures; it creates customers.

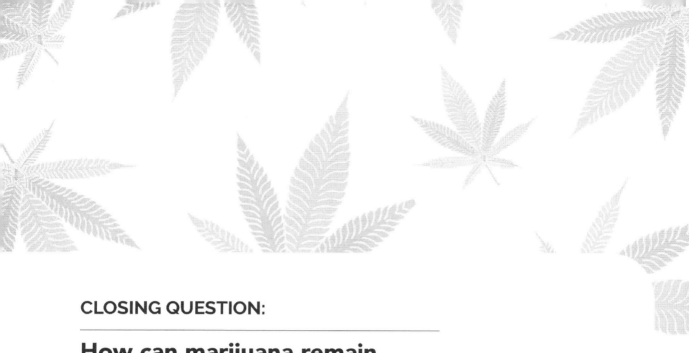

CLOSING QUESTION:

How can marijuana remain a Schedule 1 drug?

Despite the fact that it is safe and non-addictive—far more so than "harder" drugs like heroin and fentanyl—and despite the fact the government itself holds multiple patents based on the medicinal value of cannabis, the DEA refuses to acknowledge what science and society have come to accept: marijuana has no place whatsoever on the list as a Schedule 1 drug.

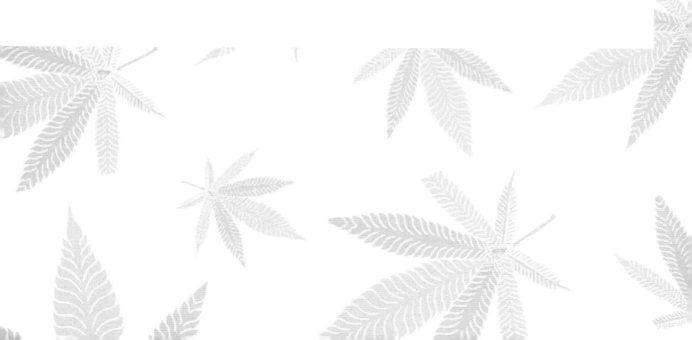

GETTING EDUCATED: THE MANY WAYS WE KNOW WEED WORKS WONDERS

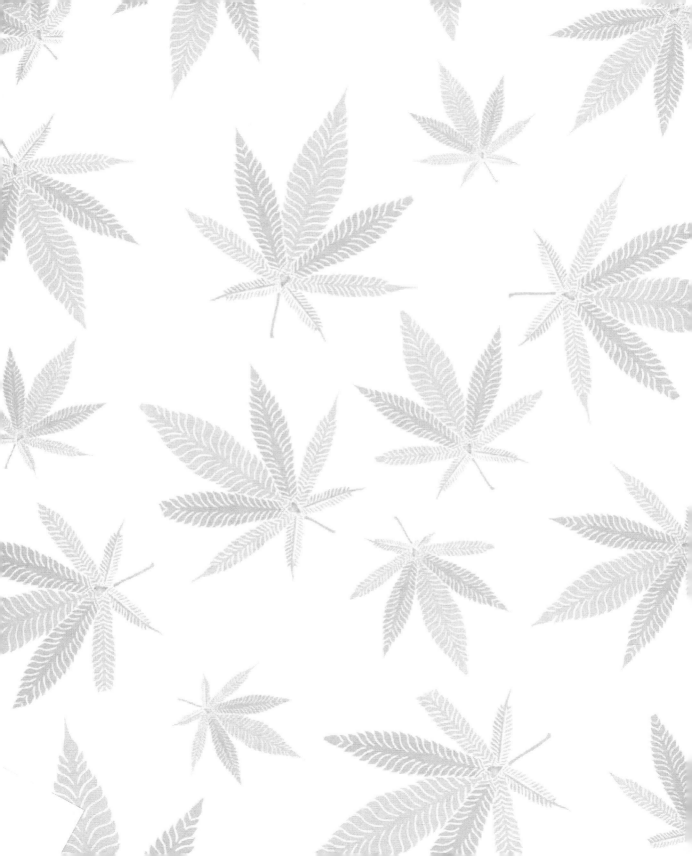

6 | SURPRISE!
YOU MIGHT
BE WRONG
ABOUT WEED

So, we're clear that we've been a bit brainwashed. Now, I'll help get you (re)educated and enlightened. Before we get into all the ways weed can work with our body and brain to help provide relief and healing, let's break down some of the most common myths and misperceptions about marijuana, shall we?

1 No, you won't find yourself an addict

Marijuana is not physically addictive. The biggest potheads can quit cold turkey with no or minimal physical effects. (By the way, nicotine, perfectly legal and readily available, is a notoriously difficult addiction to break. Alcohol withdrawals can actually kill you.) Moderate use of marijuana does not appear to pose a risk for otherwise healthy adults. Compared with alcohol or tobacco, addiction and dependency are negligible problems.

That is not to say you can't develop a habit or psychological dependency, which can be difficult to break. And, the more you use, the higher your tolerance and the more you'll need to consume to get the effect you want. Supposedly, around 9% of people who use weed heavily will become dependent on it (not physically but psychologically).

The overwhelming majority of people who do consume cannabis do not become frequent users, enjoying their weed in moderation. A 20-year epidemiological review of studies concluded that more than nine out of 10 people who use marijuana do not become dependent on the drug.

There are some people who will abuse it and take on those habits we fear: disengagement, laziness and sloth. Like anything, cannabis can be used in both healthy and unhealthy ways; but the plant itself is not addictive or dangerous. Taken intentionally and mindfully, cannabis can be used by the vast majority of people without fear of addiction or dependency.

2 You also won't end up on harder drugs

Have I beaten the "it's not a gateway drug" drum enough? Wait, one more time: it's not a gateway to anything. Claims that marijuana is a gateway to more dangerous drugs are as fanciful as the "Reefer Madness" images of murder, rape and suicide.

According to estimates from the Centers for Disease Control and Prevention, prescription opioid and heroin overdoses kill 91 Americans each day. If anything, marijuana is an exit drug. While there is zero evidence it has causal influence over harder drug use, there is growing evidence that pot is actually the path away from more harmful substances like alcohol, painkillers and tobacco. It's helping people battle their real addictions, get off harder drugs and reduce or replace their prescriptions. We'll get more into how cannabis is getting people off opioids in just a bit, but the takeaway is that it is incredibly effective.

Correlation is not causation. There is no conclusive evidence anywhere that links marijuana usage to the subsequent abuse of other illicit drugs. In fact, studies show it's alcohol and tobacco that are the actual gateways. In fact, studies show it's alcohol and tobacco that are the actual gateways. According to research from the National Institute on Drug Abuse, the overwhelming majority of people who use marijuana do not go on to use harder drugs. Meanwhile, four out of five new heroin users started off abusing prescription painkillers. The DEA has even removed the gateway theory from its website.

3 You cannot possibly overdose

Unlike opioids and harder drugs, no matter how much you consume, no amount of weed will kill you. Really. You would need to consume 1,500 pounds of marijuana in 15 minutes to be in the danger zone. It is physically impossible to die from too much marijuana. (That said, if you do get too high, you might feel like you'll die, but you won't, I assure you. I'll give you guidance in the next section on how to avoid or mitigate getting too stoned.) Marijuana doesn't interact with other drugs. There is no risk. Seriously, none.

Cannabis is the most consumed drug in the world, and yet not a single overdose has been reported. Ever. It's demonstrably safer than booze, which causes roughly six deaths every day from alcohol poisoning.

4 By the way, you don't have to get high

Just because you didn't like how you felt the last time you tried weed, doesn't mean you should shut down the idea of consumption. Cannabis has more than a hundred different chemicals that all produce different effects—the only one with psychoactivity is THC, which leaves a whole bunch of other good stuff (cannabinoids and terpenes, terms we'll get to shortly) available for you to consume without feeling altered.

Perhaps you've heard of CBD? Cannabidiol, as it's formally known, is shown to have analgesic, anti-inflammatory and anti-anxiety properties, without the psychoactive effects of THC. It is showing tremendous promise in treating people with seizures, Parkinson's, Multiple Sclerosis, Crohn's Disease and cancer, just to name a few. We'll get more into cannabis' compounds and the most promising conditions for impact shortly.

Not everyone wants to get high. In legal markets, an increasing number of options are being made available with no or low THC. While some marijuana strains are getting stronger, new ones are being developed with low THC and/or high CBD. Consumer products are being manufactured to deliver specific, targeted effects and a clear, functional high—free from lethargy, anxiety and social withdrawal. Topicals (lotions/salves and the ilk) and suppositories, even with THC in them, aren't psychoactive and won't make you loopy.

Basically, however you want to feel—or however you don't want to feel—there's a product or strain for that.

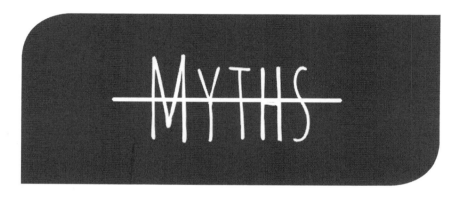

5 You also don't have to smoke a joint

If you think joints are the only way to enjoy weed, think again. They do have an old-school je ne sais quoi, which I personally enjoy; but by no means are they your only option for consumption. (By the way, I've been consuming weed for more than 20 years, and I still don't know how to roll a joint!) Have no fear; you don't have to spark up a doobie to enjoy the benefits of cannabis!

With weed's growing acceptance and its accompanying market growth, there are literally thousands of products that don't require manual dexterity or a flame. You can choose vaping, edibles, tinctures, topicals and a slew of other ways to consume without any muss, fuss or fire. (More about your options to come!) And, the accessories market is blowing up, so there's no shortage of glassware, gadgets and devices to give you whatever experience you're seeking.

Joints are still incredibly popular and fun, but if they're not your thing, your choices are many and varied. And if it's just your rolling skills at issue, you can buy pre-rolls or pre-made cones to pack yourself. Welcome to the new world of weed!

6 Weed won't destroy your lungs

As counterintuitive as it seems, lung health is hardly affected by smoking marijuana—smoking cannabis isn't the same as tobacco, other than the way in which it's consumed. There is no doubt tobacco causes lung cancer—80-90% of lung cancer cases are due to tobacco; but there is no conclusive evidence that marijuana does. In fact, not only does smoking marijuana not cause cancer, it also doesn't harm lung function. Nothing is conclusive, but what evidence we do have indicates that weed is actually beneficial to our lungs, not detrimental, as is our default assumption. In 2006 a review of research to date did not show an increase in lung cancer related to marijuana use. Many studies have proven that habitual use of marijuana does not lead to abnormalities in lung function and have found no link to negative lung health. In fact, some studies link improved lung function to long-term marijuana use. Any effects from marijuana use appear to be short-lived, resolving upon the cessation of smoking weed. Yes, really!

By the way, not only does cannabis not cause cancer, in the lab, it's been shown to actually kill cancer cells. More on that to come, stay with me! And not only does it not damage lungs, it may actually improve lung function. A bunch of studies have shown that cannabis acts as a bronchodilator, rather than a bronchoconstrictor, and enhances general lung function. Promising news for asthma, COPD and other patients who suffer with respiratory symptoms.

The damage we perceive is far worse than any actual damage to our lungs from chronic use. And where there may be issues, it's not with weed and the active ingredients of the plant, but with the combustion of plant material and the potentially toxic by-products. (There are also ways to get the benefits of cannabis without smoking it, such as vaping; read on to learn how.) So, if you enjoy blazing up, go for it (in moderation, of course). Your doctor probably won't be on board, but ultimately your health is in your control. If you make knowledgeable and informed decisions, you can make them with confidence.

7 It won't make you fat

Don't fear the munchies. First of all, not every strain makes you want to devour the contents of your kitchen or go on a Taco Bell run. (Some do, and people undergoing chemotherapy are grateful for that.) We'll get into the different strains and effects later. As it happens, THCv, one of the cannabinoids found in cannabis, is a known appetite suppressant (it's not the same as THC and not as prevalent, but it is a compound getting attention!). That said, people do tend to eat more while high—and yet, multiple studies have shown that pot smokers are thinner than our non-consuming counterparts.

That's right, regular users of marijuana have smaller waists, higher levels of good cholesterol and lower body mass index (BMI), in addition to lower incidence of diabetes. No kidding! Multiple studies have identified a reduced prevalence of obesity in the cannabis community, regardless of how or what they consume. Somehow, marijuana works to improve insulin control, regulating body weight and perhaps explaining the lower incidence of diabetes. Researchers don't yet know what it is about weed that makes it such a useful regulator of blood sugar, or how it manages to speed up metabolism, but they do know there's something to it!

8 You won't turn stupid or lazy

If you consume cannabis, your brain will not look like a fried egg, nor will your IQ be lowered. (That is not to say you might face some cognitive impairment if you overconsume, but there is no long-lasting effect.) The cannabis community has been plagued by the slothful, stupid stoner stereotype, yet recent research suggests that weed does not, indeed, make you stupid. Multiple studies confirm that cannabis doesn't destroy your brain cells, nor does it cause brain damage with long-term, heavy use. To be clear, I'm assuming you are an adult with a fully developed brain. If not, then do not pass go and do not consume—younger brains are still taking shape, and consuming cannabis while the prefrontal cortex is still developing could have repercussions later in life.

Once again surprising people with the facts, multiple studies have found that regular consumers of marijuana are more physically and socially active than non-consumers. Your short-term motivation might be impacted if you've gotten couchlock or sleepy from a particular strain or product, but generally speaking, you're not going to turn into a couch potato. You don't need to be concerned with catching amotivational syndrome or permanent couchlock.

For anyone who claims consuming cannabis kills your motivation, take a look at the entrepreneurs, activists and others within the cannabis industry who are working night and day to turn this into a legitimate, professional $20 billion business in just a few short years. We all share a special kind of motivation, willpower, passion and determination.

STILL THINK POT MAKES YOU
STUPID AND UNMOTIVATED?

Meet some other successful stoners who might surprise you:

Steve Jobs	Morgan Freeman
Rick Steves	Lily Tomlin
Carl Sagan	Jennifer Aniston
Susan Sarandon	Paul McCartney
Kathy Bates	Melissa Etheridge
Aaron Sorkin	Richard Branson
Stephen King	Neil DeGrasse Tyson
Whoopi Goldberg	*(an astrophysicist, by the way)*

"When I was a kid I inhaled frequently.
That was the point."

Barack Obama
44th President of the United States

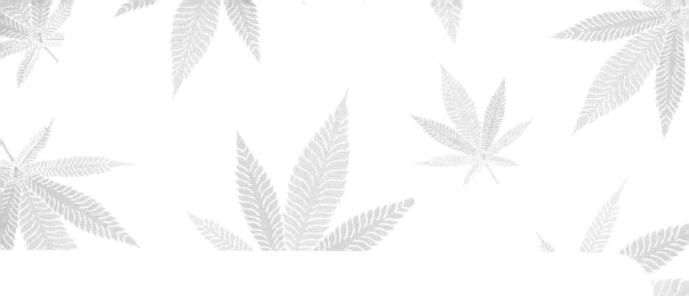

CLOSING QUESTION:

Wait—pretty much everything I feared about weed is unfounded?

Yup. The myths and misperceptions about marijuana are pervasive and pretty hard to break. Weed is not the boogeyman we've been told to fear. Even some people who believe in the medical potential of cannabis still have fears and concerns that prevent them from exploring its potential for themselves or a loved one. We've been programmed to believe things about marijuana that simply aren't true. It's time to open our eyes and wake up to the simple truth: worrying about weed is warrantless.

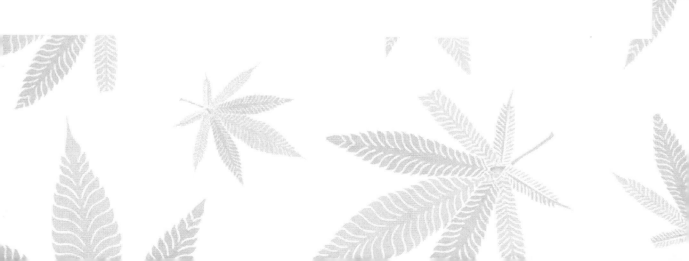

7 | GUESS WHAT? WE'RE WIRED FOR WEED!

Every human (and every animal, for that matter) has an endocannabinoid system (ECS). It is perhaps the most important, and yet least commonly known, physiological system in your body—a group of receptors distributed throughout your brain and body that are proven to play a role in everything from regulating pain, inflammation and even joint function, to sleep, appetite, anxiety and our moods. It is a part of our endocrine system and directly affects our immune, adrenal health, hormones, cellular health, mental health, pain, inflammation and nervous system. It is, quite simply, the bridge between body and mind.

The discovery of our ECS is relatively recent, which is why so few people and physicians know much, if anything, about it. It was discovered in 1992 by world-renowned researcher and Israeli biochemist, Dr. Raphael Mechoulam, the father of modern marijuana who discovered THC and CBD back in the 60s. Dr. Mechoulam identified the endogenous "bliss molecule" Anandamide and CB1 receptors in the early 1990s (CB2 receptors were found later). It became clear the human body contained a system of receptors and produced compounds very similar to those found in marijuana. Dr. Mechoulam named it the endo-cannabinoid system and thus kicked off a new generation of medical cannabis research in Israel and subsequently across the world. Many say it's a scientific breakthrough similar in magnitude to the discovery of antibodies in the 20th century.

Your ECS has billions of receptors throughout the body: in your brain, organs, connective tissue, glands and immune cells. Two primary cell receptors make up the endocannabinoid system: Cannabinoid Receptor 1 (CB1) and Cannabinoid Receptor 2 (CB2). CB1 receptors are abundant in the brain and central nervous system, white blood cells, gastrointestinal and urinary tracts, kidney, liver and lungs. CB2 receptors are also found in the brain but are also often found on immune cells, in the gastrointestinal tract and in the peripheral nervous system, which helps mitigate pain and inflammation.

These receptors bind like a lock and key with the endocannabinoids your body naturally produces (endo = produced internally). Receptors are the locks and endocannabinoids are the key. Ever had a runner's high? That's your ECS at work. Anandamide, otherwise known as the bliss molecule, is your body's own THC!

THE ENDOCANNABINOID SYSTEM

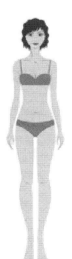

CB1 RECEPTORS

Brain/Central Nervous System
White Blood Cells
Gastrointestinal Tract
Kidneys
Liver
Lungs

CB2 RECEPTORS

Immune Support
Peripheral Nervous System
Connective Tissue

HELPS REGULATE

Appetite
Anxiety
Energy & Balance
Immune Function
Memory
Metabolism
Mood
Pain
Sleep
Temperature Regulation

Fun fact: these receptors also bind like a lock and key with the phytocannabinoids found in cannabis. See, you're actually wired for weed!

Why is Your ECS So Important?

The primary function of your endocannabinoid system is to maintain balance and stability, otherwise known as homeostasis. With receptor sites spread throughout the body, endocannabinoids are important to your day-to-day bodily function, helping regulate:

Sleep	Memory
Pain	Motor control
Appetite, digestion and hunger	Temperature regulation
Mood	Reproduction and fertility
Immune function	Pleasure and reward

A healthy and functional ECS is essential for health; it is a central component of the health and healing of every human and animal. When your endocannabinoid system is disrupted, through stress and other conditions, it can fall out of balance. Systemic stress and inflammation lead to imbalances, conditions and illness.

Many experts speculate that an ECS deficiency (Clinical Endocannabinoid Deficiency or CECD), or an imbalance in your system, is the underlying cause behind many diseases, conditions and disorders, from inflammatory and autoimmune diseases to depression, fatigue and chronic pain. The idea is simple: you are more susceptible to illness when the body does not produce enough endocannabinoids or cannot regulate them properly.

Most of the disease states related to CECD are marked by chronic pain, dysfunctional immune systems, fatigue and mood imbalances.

There is growing evidence that imbalances in the endocannabinoid system play a role in fibromyalgia, IBS and chronic migraine. These conditions display common patterns that suggest an underlying Clinical Endocannabinoid Deficiency that may be suitably treated with cannabinoid medicines. (Stay with me, we're getting into the cannabinoids next.) ECS deficiencies may play a key role in a host of other diverse neurological and otherwise seemingly unexplained illnesses.

Since the endocannabinoid system regulates most of these physiological processes and is the largest neurotransmitter system in the body, it is not surprising that these symptoms, illnesses and diseases may be caused by a deficiency in endocannabinoids. CECD may be the culprit behind these systemic physiological challenges.

Where's the Weed Come In?

Cannabis is chock-full of compounds called cannabinoids, which, like endocannabinoids, also bind like a lock and key to the CB1 and CB2 receptors throughout your ECS. These receptors are wired to bind with the endoccannabinoids your body produces naturally, or with the phytocannabinoids found within cannabis. Delta-9-tetrahydrocannabinol, or THC, is the most well-known cannabinoid, but there are more than 100 that have been identified; others such as cannabidiol (CBD), cannabinol (CBN) and cannabichromene (CBC) are gaining the interest of researchers due to a variety of healing properties.

While THC is the compound that makes you feel high and euphoric, its most important effect may be to modulate and moderate the perception of pain. Compounds that bind to the CB2 site will help with inflammation and perhaps even boost the immune system.

Now that you know about your endocannabinoid system, let's take a quick look into cannabis and how its cannabinoids do their thing.

IF MY ECS SO IMPORTANT, WHY DON'T I KNOW ABOUT IT?

The ECS was only recently discovered, despite being part of our physiology for millennia. Thank Dr. Raphael Mechoulam, the father of modern cannabis who discovered THC and CBD back in the 60s. A world-renowned researcher and chemical scientist, Dr. Mechoulam identified the endogenous "bliss molecule" Anandamide and CB1 receptors in the early 1990s (CB2 receptors were found later). It became clear the human body contained a system of receptors and compounds very similar to those found in marijuana. Dr. Mechoulam named it the endocannabinoid system and thus kicked off a new generation of medical cannabis research in Israel and subsequently across the world.

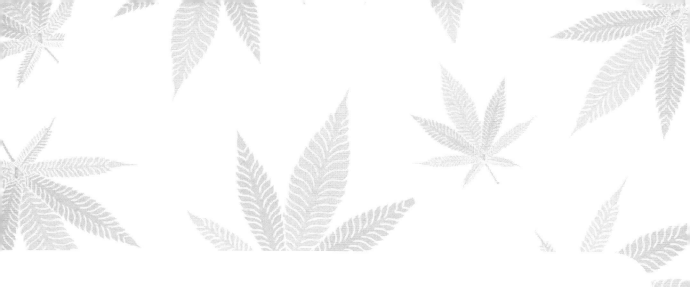

CLOSING QUESTION:

So, we all have an endocannabinoid system that regulates pretty much everything?

We do! Although we are just starting to learn about our ECS and how it works, we do know that it is a key to our physiological health and well-being. Millions of receptors throughout our brains and bodies naturally bind with the endocannabinoids that affect just about every aspect of our daily functioning. And every one of those receptors is able to bind with cannabinoids from cannabis to deliver an ever-growing number of known benefits. We are actually wired for weed!

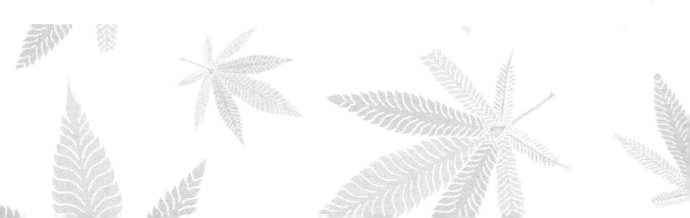

8 | THE CHEMISTRY BEHIND CANNABIS

Ok, so we've covered how your body's endocannabinoid system is responsible for balancing everything from your belly to your moods, and can be the source of—and solution to—inflammation, disease and pain. Now let's get into how cannabis and its different compounds work to deliver a range of effects and benefits.

With hundreds of chemicals making up its composition, cannabis is chock-full of cannabinoids and terpenes, which come together to form each strain's unique blueprint. Cannabinoids such as THC and CBD are what bind to your body's chemical receptors and have been shown to alleviate symptoms such as pain, nausea, seizures, and inflammation.

Terpenes, which are found in plants, fruits, herbs and spices, are what make marijuana both flavorful and pungent. If you've ever heard weed referred to as tasting like cotton candy, diesel fuel or blueberries, that's the terpene profile. That smell and aroma we all know as it wafts by? All terps. Without them, weed would have almost no taste or smell—imagine drinking a glass of wine without flavor or aroma. Not quite the same, huh? At least wine's aroma doesn't carry through doors and ventilation systems.

While science is able to isolate the individual compounds such as CBD or THC, we've also found that single cannabinoid extractions are not as effective as whole plant. Referred to as the "Entourage Effect," cannabinoids and terpenes work together to deliver a synergistic effect on body and mind. It's what distinguishes one strain from another, and is instrumental in delivering pot's physiological and psychoactive effects.

As we learn more about these various compounds and the effects different combinations produce, strains are being genetically engineered and products are being formulated and designed to help maximize medical efficacy, deliver targeted results and enable a truly customized and controllable experience.

Let's dig a little deeper into cannabinoids and terpenes!

Get to Know the Key Cannabinoids

We don't know the precise number of cannabinoids in cannabis, and most of them are at very low levels, making it difficult to accurately detect and, therefore, study them. The point is there are many, and presumably we'll learn a lot more as research opens up; for now, here's a closer look at some of the major cannabinoids you should know about.

Tetrahydrocannabinol (THC)

The most widely known cannabinoid due to its abundance and psychoactive attributes. (Psychoactive means it affects brain function and can alter perception, mood, consciousness or behavior.) Just as anandamide binds to receptors to produce a "runner's high," THC binds to those same receptors to produce that same euphoric high. Depending on how you're wired, the composition of the strain and its concentration of THC, that high could produce strong feelings of calm and peace or it could increase anxiety levels.

THC isn't just about getting high. More and more studies are coming out that bring THC's medical value to light. Multiple preclinical studies are showing that THC destroys cancer cells and kills tumors, and reverses and prevents brain damage. It helps people with PTSD. It's even been proven to have antibacterial properties in laboratory studies.

It also has another superpower: THC is a potent anti-inflammatory. Inflammation is an underlying factor behind autoimmune diseases, neurodegenerative diseases and depression.

The list of benefits is long, but here's a list of a few of the things THC specifically takes on:

Chronic and neuropathic pain	Crohn's Disease (and IBS)
Alzheimer's Disease	Arthritis
Depression	Glaucoma
Multiple Sclerosis	Insomnia
Parkinson's Disease	Stroke
PTSD	Migraines
Cancer	

Cannabidiol (CBD)

Completely nonpsychoactive, CBD is all relaxation without intoxication or cognitive impairment. Oh, and it has some serious life-saving potential.

Overlooked until recently, it's coming up hot and fast on THC, gaining perhaps its greatest recognition for stopping seizures in kids. (If you haven't watched Sanjay Gupta's *Weed* series on CNN, go watch that when you're done reading.)

This wonder cannabinoid can stop spasms, protect the brain and soothe those in chronic pain. It reduces inflammation, is an antioxidant and neuroprotectant, regulates sleep cycles and helps ease anxiety and depression. All without causing cognitive impairment.

CBD taps into the vast network of receptors throughout our endocannabinoid system (ECS) to deliver its therapeutic effects, helping with everything from neuroprotection and stress recovery, to immune balance and homeostatic regulation. It has been difficult to study, but early clinical trials, medical cannabis patients and growing anecdotal evidence point to a range of reasons to use CBD:

Chronic and neuropathic pain	Osteoporosis
Anti-inflammatory	Motor disorders
Cancer	Parkinson's Disease
Diabetes	Nicotine addiction
Depression	Psychosis & bipolar disorder
Anxiety	Epilepsy
Lupus	

So here's the interesting thing: CBD appears to counter the effect of THC 's psychoactivity. This means if you do get a little too high, some CBD will bring you back down. It also means that you can consume high-CBD/low-THC cannabis that won't get you too high, giving you the benefits of THC without the psychoactivity.

Cannabichromene (CBC)

Next in line behind CBD as the third most common cannabinoid, and also nonpsychoactive. CBC is showing to be most effective when combined with THC, CBD and other cannabinoids, fighting inflammation (particularly when combined with THC), destroying cancer tumors, relieving pain and killing bacteria. It seems to also help with brain and nerve-cell regeneration. And, it puts you in a better mood.

Cannabinol (CBN)

An analgesic that is created from the breakdown of THC through oxidization. It is mildly psychoactive and is only found in small quantities within fresh cannabis plants. In higher quantities, it can have a sedative effect (some say as effective as valium), great for treating insomnia. It is also shown to be an appetite stimulant, help with pain relief, reduce anxiety and relieve pressure behind the eyes.

Cannabigerol (CBG)

Though not prevalent in most strains, CBG might be the next big cannabinoid to hit the scene. Recent research indicates it is likely to be the "stem cell" for THC and CBD, which means that both THC and CBD start out as CBG. It's most well known for its antibacterial and pain-relief effects, and has also been found to inhibit the uptake of GABA (a neurotransmitter that blocks impulses in the brain and is linked to anxiety, pain and sleep issues), delivering a feeling of calm and ease. And, like most of the other cannabinoids, it will reduce inflammation.

Say Hello to Terpenes, You've Met Before

Let me introduce you to terpenes. You might recognize them from their scent. Weed smells for a reason, and it's all because of the terps. Love the aroma or hate it, these terpenes do more than impart taste and smell to marijuana—they are also critical components behind whatever effect cannabis delivers.

Terpenes aren't unique to cannabis, by the way. These complex organic compounds are found widely in nature, from plants and herbs to fruits and spices. When you hear someone talking about how their weed tastes like blueberries or cheese, it's not because they're already high; it's because of the terpenes. They give cannabis its diverse palate of flavors, much like you find in the world of wine.

Beyond their role in taste and flavor, terpenes interact synergistically with weed's cannabinoids to shape the feelings and effects a strain delivers. Terpenes are even being used to shape your mood; a company called LucidMood has built its entire business on the promise of what these tiny little chemicals can do. Terpenes interact with cannabinoids to create these different effects in the body, creating a unique strain profile that delivers its own set of sensory and medical aspects. You can even fine-tune your experience by figuring out which strain profile gives you the effects you're seeking.

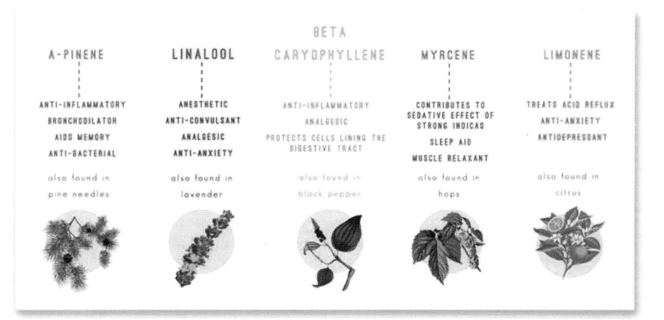

A-PINENE	LINALOOL	BETA CARYOPHYLLENE	MYRCENE	LIMONENE
ANTI-INFLAMMATORY	ANESTHETIC	ANTI-INFLAMMATORY	CONTRIBUTES TO SEDATIVE EFFECT OF STRONG INDICAS	TREATS ACID REFLUX
BRONCHODILATOR	ANTI-CONVULSANT	ANALGESIC		ANTI-ANXIETY
AIDS MEMORY	ANALGESIC	PROTECTS CELLS LINING THE DIGESTIVE TRACT	SLEEP AID	ANTIDEPRESSANT
ANTI-BACTERIAL	ANTI-ANXIETY		MUSCLE RELAXANT	
also found in	also found in	also found in	also found in	also found in
pine needles	lavender	black pepper	hops	citrus

More than 100 terpenes have been found in cannabis (over 10,000 have been identified in the plant kingdom), and we are just beginning to scratch the surface of how these diverse molecules are influencing its physiological and psychoactive effects. We do know they work in concert with cannabinoids to either catalyze or inhibit their effects. Some are especially successful in relieving stress, while others promote focus and acuity.

Myrcene with its musky, earthy aroma, for example, produces a body buzz, whereas ß-Caryophyllene, with its anise aroma, for example, increases euphoria. Citrusy whereas citrusy limonene elevates mood and kills bacteria and breast-cancer cells. Alpha-pinene is good for memory (and improving airflow to your lungs), whereas linalool helps you chill out and sleep.

The (Whole) Plant is Greater Than the Sum of its Parts

There are many mighty compounds in cannabis, as we've just broken down. However, there's this thing called the "Entourage Effect"—synergies that come from the unique inter-actions of the plant's chemical components and magnify its therapeutic benefits. Basically, while one compound is good and may deliver multiple benefits, together they create a medicinal effect where the whole is greater than the sum of the parts. Isolating compounds such as THC or CBD diminishes their power and potential.

Myrcene can reduce resistance in the blood-brain barrier to help other chemicals break through. Pinene helps counteract the spacey-ness caused by THC. THC plus CBN will knock you out, if you need to sleep or chill out. A 1:1 ratio of THC:CBD is the perfect balance for a clear, functional high without the side effects like anxiety that many people fear. The combinations are endless, we are just beginning to scratch the surface of what's possible.

Caution Jumping on the CBD-Only Bandwagon

CBD is amazing, don't get me wrong. Its results have driven a media frenzy. Have you heard of Charlotte Figi? We saw her go from 300 seizures per week to just one on Dr. Sanjay Gupta's CNN *Weed* documentary. Charlotte lives in Colorado and was using a high-CBD, low-THC strain that has become known today as Charlotte's Web.

People went searching the internet for this "miracle oil." The void quickly filled with both legit and shady businesses. Hemp-derived CBD is legal, but that doesn't mean the end product is safe or effective. The quality of input—whole plant or just stems and stalks; and the quality of output—how it's processed and produced, are important factors.

For many, given legal limitations, hemp-derived CBD is the only option. (Remember that hemp is the variation of cannabis with almost no THC.) There are plenty of quality producers. But, beware the snake oil. Unlike the highly regulated marijuana market, hemp-derived CBD falls under the FDA's purview as a nutritional supplement. No guidelines. No regulations. No review of safety or effectiveness. It has, however, issued a warning about firms claiming their product contains CBD when it doesn't, and warned consumers about unsubstantiated medical claims. (You can find a list of red flagged firms on the FDA's website.)

What's most important is the quality of the product and the processing. Cannabis cannot be certified as organic, but you should confirm the plant was grown without pesticides and other harmful chemicals. Look for products produced in a GMP facility and that offer testing results—regulations vary state to state, there is no standard; but reputable companies will provide assurance of quality.

In states where cannabis is legally available, products derived from the marijuana plant (versus hemp) can offer better and more options for CBD products. In a regulated market, you'll find stringent testing. Many producers are focusing on high-CBD/low-THC strains and products like edibles and concentrates, often with far higher concentrations of CBD than in hemp-derived products.

And, if you've been hung up on those three little letters—THC—stop. Please. One more time: you don't have to get high to reap the full benefits available through the whole plant.

Coming (Back) Out of the Closet

Cannabis is essentially a natural pharmacy, and can be a most useful tool in treating—and even preventing—a wide variety of diseases and conditions. Our bodies are wired for it, for crying out loud! It was a component of healing for indigenous civilizations across the planet, and is slowly regaining recognition for its efficacy as a medicine.

From the painkilling, tumor-destroying effects of THC to the anti-inflammatory, antispasmodic benefits of CBD, we have just begun to scratch the surface of what's possible. Researchers are digging deeper and people are waking up; we are at the dawn of a new way to wellness.

I'm hopeful for a future where cannabis-based medicines have a place in the worldwide pharmacopeia again. Where researchers can study and document its far-reaching benefits. And where people can access the healing and enhancing properties of the plant with ease and confidence.

One day, future generations will look back and wonder how these dark ages of dank could have endured for so long.

WEED FOR YOUR PET

CBD can help pets feel and function better, too. They also have an endocannabinoid system (ECS), and so can benefit from many of the same effects CBD delivers to the body, canine or feline. It can help with everything from arthritis and compromised immune systems, to stress responses, aggression and digestive issues. It can also be useful in treating acute issues like sprains and breaks and even during post-operative care to reduce swelling, pain and stiffness.

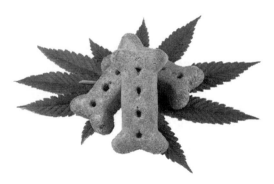

As with all your loved ones, you want to put good things into their bodies. Do your homework, ask your vet and make sure the product you buy is made well and isn't on the FDA's flagged list.

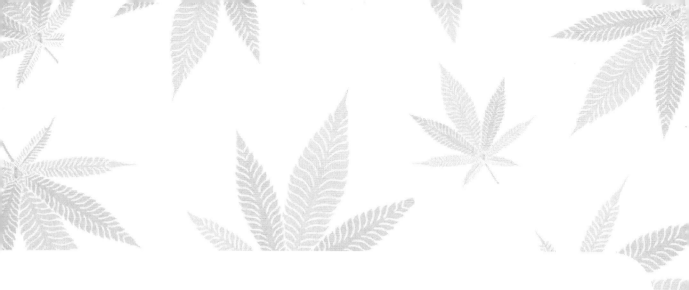

CLOSING QUESTION:

Weed isn't just about THC? And THC isn't just about getting you high?

Nope! Cannabis has hundreds of compounds that are just being discovered and explored—CBD and a handful of other cannabinoids are showing substantive and credible promise in taking on a wide range of conditions and illnesses. Terpenes take weed's effects in a range of directions. And THC does so much more than get you high without requiring that you actually get high, so don't take it off the table. Don't forget, while each compound is mighty in its own way, the magic really happens when they all work together.

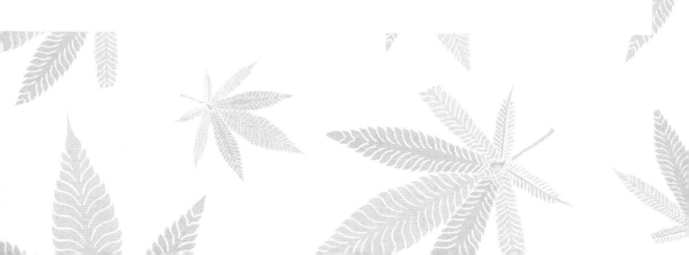

9 | ON POT AND PAINKILLERS...

Marijuana is medicine.

By now that should be obvious. Perhaps nowhere can this be more impactful than with the opioid epidemic faced in our country. Cannabis has the potential to be the single biggest answer to what could be the single biggest health crisis our country faces.

Headlines abound with tragic stories of people losing their lives—literally or figuratively—to opioids. Prescription painkillers are more widely used than tobacco. Drug deaths in America are rising faster than ever. Nearly 60,000 people lost their lives to overdose in 2016, an increase of nearly 20% over 2015. It's is the leading cause of accidental death in the U.S., with 20,101 deaths related to prescription pain relievers in 2015 alone.

The epidemic kicked off in the 1990s, when overprescribing began for chronic pain. It seems pharmaceutical companies reassured the medical community that patients would not become addicted to prescription opioid pain relievers, and healthcare providers began to prescribe them at greater rates. Big Pharma knew they were wrong, but, hey, there was a market to penetrate.

A recent Harvard study confirms Big Pharma exploited the enormous addiction potential of opioids to prey upon the American populace for decades—enabled by a federal government with non-rigorous patenting standards and ineffectual policing of companies using fraudulent marketing. The cozy relationship between Big Pharma and government has grown, with the pharmaceutical industry spending close to $2.5 billion dollars in ten years on lobbying federal and state governments and campaign contributions. It outspends other industries by far on lobbying—90% of the House and 97% of the Senate have taken contributions from Big Pharma.

NOT-FUN FACTS ABOUT AMERICA'S OPIOID CRISIS

Since 1999, opioid overdose **deaths have quadrupled.**

We consume **80% of the world's opioids,** yet are only 4% of the world's population.

99% of the world's hydrocodone is consumed in the United States.

As of 2016, more than **289 million prescriptions** were written per year.

35% of adults were prescribed painkillers in 2016.

2 million abuse prescription painkillers.

More than **90 people die** every day after overdosing on opioids.

Opioid abuse **costs ~$72 million** a year.

Every 3 minutes, a woman goes to the emergency room for abuse or misuse of prescription painkillers.

From 2008-2012, substance abuse **admissions increased by 70%** for those 50+.

The crisis is hitting close to home for women. Since 1999, overdose deaths from prescription painkillers are up 400 percent, nearly twice as high as the rate for men. And for every overdose, 30 women go to the emergency room for painkiller misuse or abuse.

Oh, by the way, women are more likely to have chronic pain, be prescribed prescription painkillers, be given higher doses and use them for longer time periods than men. And seniors have prescriptions thrown at them by the dozens (14 to be exact), for everything from post-surgical pain to arthritis, to chronic back pain or a strain from a golf swing. Fifty-five million opioid prescriptions were written in 2016 for people 65+—a 20% increase in the past five years. Pain clinics are an entire industry.

We all have pain at some point in our lives, and when it becomes medical-grade, we generally get prescribed an opioid painkiller. Percocet, Vicodin, OxyContin and the deadly fentanyl are all in this class of drugs, the most prescribed class of medications in the United States. Used for short periods, addiction is generally a non-issue. But lots of people don't want to take an opioid at all, for any length of time; others are simply unable to safely take pain medication because of interaction, reaction or past addiction issues—and so they are left to suffer. And, over longer periods of time, chronic usage can become problematic, even if it's not an addiction.

Overprescribing continues, despite no real proof that opioids actually do anything for the third of the population suffering from chronic pain. For those of us who suffer from it, little is known about rates of addiction. Personally, I don't see how you don't develop a dependency on opioids after an extended period of use, regardless of your addictive or non-addictive tendencies. They create physical dependency and need for increased use over time. It's a pretty simple, but sad, premise.

But here's where the data start to back up how much of an impact cannabis can have: multiple studies have shown that in states where medical marijuana has been legalized, there are fewer prescriptions written, far fewer opioid addictions and fewer deaths—25% less, in fact. According to a new study in the journal *Drug and Alcohol Review*, people are increasingly substituting cannabis for prescription medication, alcohol, and illicit drugs, the majority (80.6%) forgoing pharmaceuticals for the non-toxic alternative.

And of particular relevance to me, and perhaps to you or someone you love, researchers found that women over the age of 40 showed the most significant decrease in problematic painkiller use.

Weed works. Really. I'm a woman over 40 who is no longer a problematic painkiller user.

MY PERSONAL CONNECTION WITH PERCOCET

I am one of the millions who was prescribed opioids (percocet to be exact, and a lot of it) for chronic pain. For nearly three years, I struggled to manage pain when over-the-counter products were not an option for me. (Except Tylenol, which is like taking a Tic-Tac, and will destroy your liver and can be toxic.) My tolerance increased, and so did the quantity and dosage prescribed. I hated how I felt. It was like living under a lead blanket. I was depressed and disengaged in life.

By the time I left New York for Colorado, where medical marijuana is legal, I was taking 180 pills a month. And it was barely working; my pain management doctor told me my only option was to step up to a more potent opioid. Um, no thanks. I was on the verge of a serious addiction, and was at a fork in the road. I could keep going down the rabbit hole or go full stop.

I went full stop. Since the move, I'm off the pills entirely for my chronic pain. I could not have done it without cannabis to ease the withdrawal symptoms and to manage the chronic pain going forward.

I am far from the only success story of how weed can help people wean themselves off a deadly and addictive drug. Individual stories and research studies continue to come out in support of marijuana's effectiveness in battling the painkiller epidemic.

But it's not just about problematic use or addiction; it's about an alternative. One that is safer and with fewer side effects. One that improves the quality of life for millions.

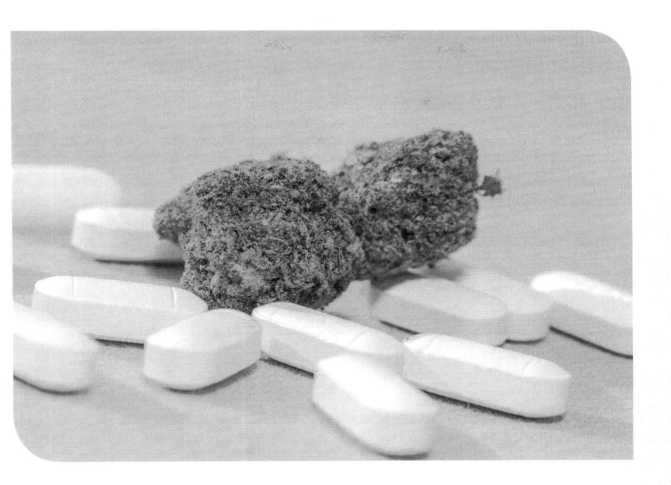

How Can Pot Possibly Replace or Reduce Painkillers?

Millions of people are finding pot to be a better, more preferable alternative to prescription painkillers. Physicians have commented for more than a century on the potential for cannabis to substitute for opioid drugs, and multiple recent studies are proving this to be true. While clinical studies are lagging because of Schedule 1 research constraints, the evidence mounts daily of weed's efficacy in treating pain.

Numerous studies have proven the effectiveness of cannabis as a pain reliever, in addition to a slew of other therapeutic benefits. It is also becoming the preferred alternative for alcohol, drugs and prescriptions by many. Beyond the federal Medicare and Medicaid data showing drastic reductions in prescriptions in states where medical marijuana is available (4-5X reductions for painkillers), people are self-reporting through surveys and other studies that they are finding as much, if not more, relief from cannabis as they do from painkillers. They're also reporting no or limited side effects, as well as better quality of life and better mood.

Marijuana also acts as an amplifier, so to speak, for opioids. A little cannabis can significantly augment the analgesic effects of painkillers. Technically called a co-agonist, each magnifies the effect of the other—which means you can take a lower dose of narcotics and still have it be effective. The combination of the two can bring pain levels down using smaller amounts of opioids for shorter periods of time.

Simply put, pot is good for pain. And it's not just good, it's safe. No matter how you look at it, the benefits far outweigh the risks. You can't overdose, addiction is a minimal risk, it has far fewer side effects than opioids and it improves quality of life. The latest line from our government with regards to opioids is to "just say no." That isn't much of a solution, but saying "yes" to cannabis just may be.

66 The real story is the hypocrisy around medical marijuana. People think it's a gateway drug to narcotics. It may be the exit drug to get us out of the narcotic epidemic. 99

DR. MEHMET OZ
Physician, TV Host, Author
(said while on an appearance on FOX News)

HOW DOES WEED WORK ON YOUR BRAIN?

If you recall your lesson on our endocannabinoid system (ECS) and the chemistry of cannabis, THC binds to CB1 receptors in the brain and central nervous system. While it doesn't actually eliminate the pain, it works with your brain to make you less aware and focused on it. It takes the edge off, so to speak. And since CB1 receptors are not in the part of the brain that regulates heart rate and respiration, unlike narcotics, there isn't a lethal dose; someone can consume as much is needed for its palliative effects.

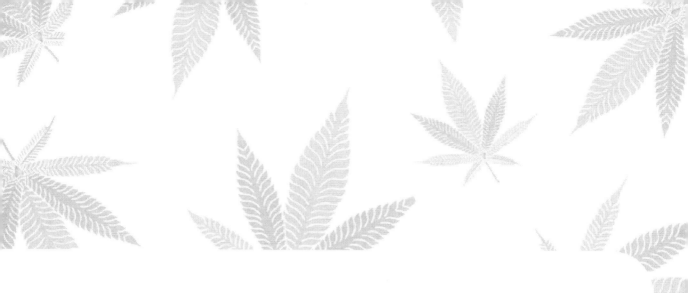

CLOSING QUESTION:

So for someone with chronic pain, cannabis can be a safe and effective way to manage it?

That is correct! With none of the risks or side effects found with painkillers, like overdose and addiction, weed is a really good option for many people. It is natural and safe, with limited to no side effects (all of which are controllable). Cannabis is helping millions break their dependencies and improve the quality of their lives. Could it help you or someone you love?

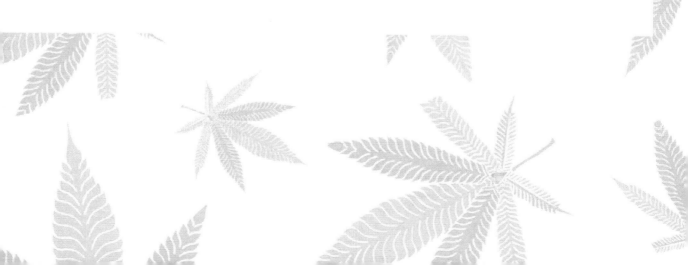

10 | WEED, WORKING ITS MAGIC ON A WIDE RANGE OF CONDITIONS...

Healers have used cannabis to treat illnesses, maladies and disease for thousands of years. This plant really is the jack-of-all-trades when it comes to relief. Or perhaps better said, *releaf*.

The number of conditions that weed may treat is vast and growing as more research becomes available. For many, cannabis offers a real possibility for natural relief that could replace (or reduce) multiple prescriptions. To recap our earlier lesson: it has no risk of overdose and side effects and drug interactions are minimal and manageable (but should be monitored).

Here's a shortlist of top issues people are using cannabis to treat:

Anxiety

Not everyone can treat anxiety with cannabis. For some, smoking pot causes acute anxiety and paranoia, but that effect is often connected with the type of marijuana consumed. We'll get into the weeds later, but some strains of marijuana (sativas and high-THC) can induce anxiety (especially for newbies), whereas others (indicas) can deliver strong relaxation and anxiety reduction properties.

When it comes to anxiety, THC and CBD can have the opposite effects: THC can create paranoia and anxiety in some, because it activates the amygdala area of the brain, which is responsible for fear. And recall that CBD counteracts the effects of THC. On its own, CBD can lower—even eliminate—anxiety.

Chances are, if you've had a bad experience in the past with feeling anxious or paranoid, you were mismatched with your marijuana. If chilling out is on your agenda, the right strain of cannabis (1:1 ratio of THC:CBD or high CBD) can pretty much deliver all the effects of a Xanax or Valium without the side effects or interactions. In the next section, I'll give you some guidance to help identify the strains best for relieving anxiety. It's not all education— you get tools, too!

Arthritis

One out of every five adults experiences some sort of arthritis pain, and as we get older age-related osteoarthritis becomes a chronic condition for many. Cannabis helps relieve that pain both in the joints and in the brain, while it also calms the immune system and fights inflammation.

For patients with rheumatoid arthritis (RA), it seems they have an unusually high number of CB2 receptors, which means an unusually high number of sites for cannabis to fight inflammation and pain. Both CBD and THC engage with CB2 receptors. They work in different ways: THC directly connects with the receptor, triggering an anti-inflammatory response; whereas CBD increases the amount of endocannabinoids in the body, tapping into our own system of self-repair. Cannabis calms inflammation and reins in the immune system, giving nerves and tissue time to recover. Weed can also help RA patients with related symptoms like chronic fatigue, insomnia and gastrointestinal issues.

Weed works with osteoarthritis in an entirely different way, yet again demonstrating its versatility and polypharmaceutical qualities. While RA is an autoimmune disease, osteoarthritis is a degenerative disease tied to aging and excessive wear and tear, afflicting seniors and aging adults with chronic pain, stiffness and loss of flexibility. The loss of cartilage is the primary culprit behind osteoarthritis, and is irreversible and untreatable with medications. While regrowing cartilage is still a distant possibility, multiple studies are showing that cannabis protects against bone loss and slows the destruction of cartilage.

It's possible that cannabis can be a long-term alternative to prescription and over-the-counter painkillers, anti-inflammatories, corticosteroids and other medications, easing pain and reducing swelling without the potentially life-threatening side effects caused by frequent NSAID or opiate use.

Asthma/Bronchial Conditions

As contradictory as it seems, cannabis smoke doesn't impair lung function: it may actually improve it. While on the surface an unlikely medical treatment for a respiratory condition, cannabis may have beneficial effects for those with asthma or other respiratory conditions—even when smoked.

Asthma is a chronic inflammatory disease and cannabis is a known anti-inflammatory. If you'll recall, some of the cannabinoids in weed are bronchodilators, which means that they help lungs expand and take in more air. Perhaps surprisingly, THC dilates respiratory passages and inhibits coughing. Turns out, cannabis actually does the opposite of tobacco smoke in that it expands rather than constricts bronchial passageways. Studies of long-term pot users show improved lung capacity (perhaps from the huge drags we take) and efficiency. Tobacco smokers, no surprise, lost lung function.

Doctors have been surprised to see their patients get almost immediate relief from asthma attacks after smoking cannabis. The response can be as effective as the most commonly prescribed inhalers, but without the complications of corticosteroids, which can include high blood pressure, anxiety and depression, among other severe side effects.

And remember, you don't have to smoke cannabis to get its benefits. We'll get into the different options for consumption later, but there's this thing called a vaporizer, and it's a great alternative to smoking. Read on!

Autism

Parents of children with severe autism, frustrated with the lack of options, are increasingly turning to cannabis. Many have heard anecdotal reports of success; others have read of promising results with epileptic children. There are no clinical studies on cannabis and autism, but there is a growing body of positive anecdotal evidence from doctors and parents that cannabis is making children with autism happier and healthier.

There are astonishingly few approved medical treatments for autism. Only two medications have been approved by the FDA to treat the symptoms of autism: both are antipsychotic drugs that are not always effective and carry serious side effects. Anecdotal evidence indicates that CBD is helping children in ways no other medication has. Clinical trials are underway in Israel with promising results. Although too early to reach conclusions, many children have shown significant improvements. Some no longer hurt themselves or throw tantrums. Some are more communicative.

Most doctors are not willing to recommend cannabis to treat autism. There simply aren't enough data or studies; and there is legitimate concern over cannabis' impact on a developing brain. But for some families who've exhausted their options, medical marijuana or even hemp-based CBD could be a miracle treatment for their children.

Brain Disease (including Alzheimer's) and Trauma

Cannabis holds great promise in slowing, and perhaps ultimately preventing, the progression of Alzheimer's disease. The THC in cannabis destroys the plaque that causes loss of brain function; if the plaque never forms, Alzheimer's does not develop. In contrast, CBD appears to generate new brain cell growth. Plus, it reduces inflammation and alleviates symptoms like anxiety and depression.

Recall earlier I referenced the government holds patent #6630507 on CBD. It's based on the claim that "cannabinoids are found to be neuroprotectants following stroke and trauma or in the treatment of neurodegenerative diseases, such as Alzheimer's disease, Parkinson's disease and dementia."

The compounds in cannabis may decrease damage from head and brain trauma, strokes, oxygen deprivation and neurodegenerative diseases. Weed's neuroprotectants have many functions, including preventing stress-related damage and reducing inflammation in the brain.

Cannabis holds great promise for those who suffer from traumatic brain injury. In a way, compounds in cannabis are like internal shock absorbers, checking back the damage sustained with a concussion and other forms of head trauma. Whether from too many hits on the football field or the result an accident or stroke, the brain seems to be better off on weed; protecting the brain ahead of or just at the time of injury and possibly even repairing damage.

Cancer

Nearly 40% of us will be diagnosed with cancer at some point. Almost everyone is touched by it in some way. By now, most everyone accepts that cannabis is a powerful tool and amazing medicine for many cancer and treatment-related side effects such as nausea, vomiting, loss of appetite, pain, depression, anxiety and insomnia. Oncologists, more than any doctors, support cannabis as part of a treatment program for patients suffering from cancer.

People suffering terribly from their cancer treatment find great relief in weed. The THC in marijuana can help relieve pain and nausea, reduce inflammation and can act as an antioxidant. Cannabidiol (CBD) can help treat seizures, can reduce anxiety and paranoia, and can counteract the "high" caused by THC. Some people can even reduce their pain medication. And in this case, the munchies are most certainly a good thing for people who struggle to find a hint of an appetite.

Relief is good. But what is particularly exciting is cannabis' promise in actually attacking and preventing cancer. Accumulating medical research from around the world shows positive results and potential in treating brain tumors, lymphomas and cancers affecting the breast, prostate, lung, uterus, cervix, mouth, colon, biliary tract, thyroid, pancreas, skin and more.

THC and other cannabinoids cut off a tumor's blood supply, which can inhibit or stop the growth of cancers from spreading or growing. Their anti-inflammatory activity blocks cell growth, prevents the growth of blood vessels that supply tumors, fights viruses, and relieves muscle spasms. And, they also appear to activate the self-destruct function built into tumors. Called apoptosis, it's the programmed death of cancer cells. It means marijuana has the ability to target cancer cells while leaving healthy cells intact—unlike radiation and chemotherapy which kill cancer cells along with all the healthy cells surrounding them, debilitating the patient in the process It's like natural chemotherapy, without the toxic stuff that makes you sick and miserable.

While the positive effects of using cannabis to alleviate cancer symptoms have been well documented, it remains classified as a Schedule I drug with high potential for abuse (again, not!) and no known medical use (wrong, and now you know it!). Consequently, the federal government's position on cannabis stifles much-needed research on cannabis as a "cure" for cancer. Paradoxically, the federally funded National Cancer Institute has warmed up to cannabis as a cancer treatment and has even quietly acknowledged its cancer-killing properties in early clinical trials. The research is promising, but we are still a long way off from knowing if cannabis can provide a "cure."

Crohn's Disease/Colitis

There's no getting around it: Crohn's and other inflammatory bowel diseases (IBD) are awful for those who suffer from it—urgent bathroom runs, pain and cramping are regular issues. The primary culprit is inflammation in the gastrointestinal (GI) tract, which triggers most of the worst symptoms and causes abdominal pain, diarrhea, tiredness, loss of weight and malnutrition.

There is no cure for Crohn's. Many conventional Crohn's drugs seek to reduce inflammation and suppress the immune system, which is continually attacking the gut. But, many Crohn's patients don't respond to conventional treatments or have trouble managing the severe side effects of immunosuppressant drugs. A common treatment is corticosteroids, but they present a smorgasbord of side effects, from minor (hair loss) to life threatening (lowered immune response, elevated blood pressure and blood sugar levels).

If you've been paying attention, you'll recall that cannabinoids, particularly CBD, are effective anti-inflammatory agents. And, cannabinoid receptors are found throughout the GI tract and are specifically found on immune cells. Although the anti-inflammatory properties of medical cannabis hold true for all people, IBD patients have more cannabinoid receptors in their gut than people without IBD, which means they are likely to respond to the anti-inflammatory properties of medical marijuana. Studies are showing that weed serves an important purpose in treating and alleviating the symptoms of painful inflammatory bowel disorders. In addition to relieving pain, muscle cramps, anxiety, insomnia and inflammation; it can also promote appetite, produce weight gain and enhance the mood of affected patients. Ultimately, people enjoy better quality of life, greater ability to work a normal job, increased ability to perform daily tasks and maintain a social life, as well as a drastic decrease in pain reduction and mental anguish. All without accompanying side effects.

Depression

Nearly 15 million people suffer from depression; for many, it can be debilitating and destructive. It is the leading cause of disability in the United States and yet is wildly misunderstood by most.

Depression and chronic stress go hand in hand. Stress leads to chronic inflammation and imbalance of the endocannabinoid system (ECS). Endocannabinoids help balance mood and influence our reward-seeking behavior; and regulate sleep, appetite and certain aspects of the immune system. Ultimately, the ECS is what maintains balance and stability in the body.

It seems chronic stress-induced depression creates a deficiency of endocannabinoids— which can be balanced by ingesting phytocannabinoids from marijuana, thereby balancing mood and alleviating depression. Both THC and CBD are known to exert sedative, antidepressant and antipsychotic effects. In low doses, THC can serve as an antidepressant and produce serotonin—but it should be noted that high doses of THC could worsen depression symptoms.

Multitudes of patients and studies have found that cannabis helps treat depression with less-serious side effects (and more quickly) than antidepressants. It enhances mood, provides energy and focus, relieves anxiety, induces hunger and combats insomnia. People who use cannabis are generally less depressed than non-users; moderate use of cannabis appears to alleviate stress and stabilize moods. Stay away from heavy use and high-THC products, and a natural remedy might be available.

Epilepsy

Cannabis has been used to treat seizures for thousands of years, but it is only recently that we're getting the evidence to prove it. I mentioned Charlotte Figi and her miraculous response to CBD on CNN's *Weed* documentary back in 2013. Since then, the floodgates have opened in terms of interest and support from the media, the public and product developers as families seek viable solutions for their loved ones. Sixteen states now have laws that specifically allow the use of CBD to treat seizures. (Israel has officially approved CBD for the treatment of intractable pediatric epilepsy, by the way.)

We are, for the first time, getting scientific data and validation of CBD's potential to help reduce or eliminate seizures. Rigorous studies are clearly establishing CBD as an anti-seizure drug. There is recent excitement over a new CBD-based drug undergoing FDA-approved clinical trials because it has been shown to reduce convulsive seizures in children with a severe form of epilepsy by nearly half, and for 5%, stop them completely. (There were side effects, which caused some to drop out; these included drowsiness, fatigue, diarrhea and reduced appetite, similar to those caused by other epilepsy drugs.) And, while not scientific data, research in Australia revealed 71% of parents/guardians found cannabis products successful in helping manage their child's seizures; 51% reduced use of anti-epileptic drugs after introducing cannabis.

It's not clear precisely how CBD works. It appears to attach to brain cells and dampen the electrical activity; a unique mechanism of action that's not shared by any existing seizure medications. While CBD should not be viewed as a panacea for epilepsy, there is most certainly hope that we may soon have another treatment option.

For 3,800 years, healers and physicians have been prescribing cannabis and documented that use to treat epilepsy. But it's only now that we finally have the early proof that cannabis can work to treat epilepsy.

Fibromyalgia

Marijuana is outpacing prescription drugs when it comes to fibromyalgia relief. For the nearly five million Americans who suffer from fibromyalgia—a poorly understood disorder characterized by deep tissue pain, fatigue, headaches, depression and lack of sleep—options are limited. The FDA has approved only three drugs for its treatment, and although they generate billions of dollars in annual sales, most patients say they don't work.

A survey by the National Pain Foundation found that medical marijuana is far more effective at treating symptoms than any of the three prescription drugs available. Of cannabis-consuming fibromyalgia patients, 62% found marijuana "very effective" in relieving pain. Weed drastically outperformed common prescription drugs like Cymbalta, Lyrica and Savella where only 8–10% found them "very effective" in controlling symptoms. Remember when I said earlier that Big Pharma isn't happy about weed? Here's just one more reason why. It just works better for many.

If you recall your lesson on the endocannabinoid system earlier, there's a thing called Clinical Endocannabinoid Deficiency (CECD) where your system gets thrown out of whack and creates issues with mood, sleep, pain, fatigue, gastrointestinal issues and muscle spasticity. Sounds a lot like fibromyalgia, right? It's believed to be part of CECD.

How does cannabis help? THC reduces the hypersensitivity to pain experienced by fibromyalgia patients by filling in for our own body's natural endocannabinoid, anandamide. Cannabis can put an end to muscle spasms, tightness and twitching, and help get a good night's rest with deep, uninterrupted sleep. It takes on depression and nausea, and generally improves quality of life and overall physical functioning.

Glaucoma

Affecting roughly 60 million people worldwide, glaucoma is the second leading cause of blindness and is the result of progressive optic nerve damage. The root cause for the majority of glaucoma is hypertension of the eye. This intraocular pressure (IOP) initially causes the loss of peripheral vision; left untreated it can lead to blindness. And, I hate to tell you, it increases in frequency with age.

It has no cure; the process can only be slowed, or in rare cases, halted. The treatment is to somehow get the pressure down. And sadly, the vast majority of treatments require drugs that have harsh side effects or which are simply ineffective.

But, it just so happens one of the many virtues of this plant is its ability to decrease intraocular pressure. We've just discovered CB1 and CB2 receptors located directly in the tissue of the eyes, with CB1 highest in density in the mechanism that regulates IOP. It has been definitively demonstrated, and is widely appreciated, that smoking marijuana lowers IOP in both normal individuals and in those with glaucoma. These depressurizing effects of marijuana may delay the progression of glaucoma, postponing or preventing vision loss. Now that's some powerful medicine.

Insomnia

Lots of people use weed to help them sleep—in many ways, it's the ultimate sleep aid, facilitating a speedy, uninterrupted, deep and dreamless slumber. Its effects have been compared to lithium (without the drooling, for the most part!) Studies and anecdotal reports suggest that it is safer and similarly effective at treating insomnia than prescription drugs such as Ambien. And it affects sleep across its various stages and waves.

The THC in weed helps you fall asleep faster, wake up less in the first half of the night and generally sleep longer. Something that generally benefits us all. But those with sleeping disorders such as apnea, insomnia and night terrors could benefit the most. Studies have shown a dramatic reduction in sleep disturbances: people are less likely to wake up early after toking up and more likely to have a better and full night's sleep.

Be warned, it can work in reverse if weed is abruptly stopped. Heavy users who abruptly stop using marijuana report strange dreams, insomnia and poor sleep quality. And, too much THC could make you a bit foggy the next day. It's like a weed hangover.

Not only do you sleep faster and harder in the first half of your night, if you're a regular midnight toker, you will be dream-free. Cannabis before bed reduces the time spent in REM, which means you won't have as many dreams or as vivid dreams.

Oh, and fun fact, marijuana users report negligible use of alcohol, sleeping pills or other medicines to sleep. I didn't participate in the study, but can back that up. I haven't taken a sleeping pill in years and I sleep like a baby.

WHY CANNABIS CAN
COMBAT SO MANY CONDITIONS

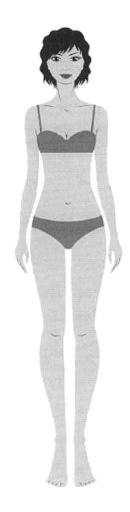

ANXIETY

CBD can reduce anxiety

ASTHMA/COPD

Cannabinoids are
bronchodialators

CANCER

THC relieves pain & nausea;
can destroy cancer cells

DEPRESSION

THC and CBD can act as
anti-depressants and help
with sleep

FIBROMYALGIA

THC relieves nerve pain

INSOMNIA

THC helps with a faster, longer
and uninterrupted sleep

MULTIPLE SCLEROSIS

THC and CBD reduce muscle
spasms

PARKINSON'S

May provide tremor relief

ARTHRITIS

CBD and THC reduce pain
and inflammation

BRAIN DISEASE

THC destroys plaque; CBD
generates new brain cells
and protects brain

CROHN'S/COLITIS

CBD is an anti-inflammatory

EPILEPSY

CBD is an anti-seizure

GLAUCOMA

Decreases intraocular
pressure

LYME DISEASE

THC is an anti-bacterial; can
help manage symptoms

PAIN

THC relieves pain; CBD is an
anti-inflammatory

WEIGHT MANAGEMENT

May reduce blood
sugar and BMI

PTSD

Cannabinoids deactivate
traumatic memories

Lyme Disease

According to the CDC, Lyme disease is the fastest growing vector-borne infectious disease in the United States. It has been found in all 50 states, and around the world. Antibiotics are the prescribed treatment, despite no evidence they cure the disease and upwards of a 40% relapse rate. It is often misdiagnosed, with an array of symptoms and manifestations that could seem like MS, chronic fatigue, lupus or depression. Or, if you've been following along, a lot like Clinical Endocannabinoid Deficiency syndrome (CEDS).

Cannabis can be used to manage the symptoms of Lyme: the pain, inflammation, fatigue from bad sleep, loss of appetite and anxiety. But it's also showing promise for some in actually eradicating it entirely. Though evidence is anecdotal, the antibacterial benefits of THC may help people make a full recovery. High concentrations of high-THC cannabis oils are being used to eliminate the bacteria that causes Lyme disease from the body and reverse the long-term damage to the nervous and immune system. It is not a recognized nor studied treatment, but for some, cannabis a last resort that is actually viable.

Multiple Sclerosis

Few conditions are as enduring and progressively debilitating as MS, which causes damage to the brain and spinal cord, and affects the body's immune system. It hits close to home for many of us, affecting millions worldwide. Patients with MS face an insurmountable amount of pain on a daily basis. A constant attack on the central nervous system means they slowly lose their ability to move their muscles and limbs. Vision and other bodily functions are also affected. There is no cure.

Treatments typically involve powerful drugs that aim to slow progression of the disease, manage symptoms and accelerate recovery after attacks. This is where cannabis comes in. Cannabis has been wildly successful in providing much-needed relief from pain, gastrointestinal distress, muscle spasms and even paralysis. People get physically better; they have greater physical activity levels, strength, speed, and less fatigue.

Cannabis is approved in 20 countries for spasms in multiple sclerosis. Significant evidence suggests THC and CBD-based medications can be used for treating muscle spasticity associated with multiple sclerosis (most studies have focused on synthetic derivative; few have examined whole-plant cannabis or many of the other MS associated symptoms). Even so, it protects the brain and helps with pain, sleep, inflammation, muscle spasms and stomach and mood issues.

As with other diseases that affect our endocannabinoid system, MS throws it out of whack. We now know that the ECS plays a crucial role in mediating symptoms of MS—cannabinoids tap into our ECS to slow down the autoimmune reaction, stop inflammation, improve muscular control and eliminate bodily side effects of MS. They also help control spasticity.

There is ample evidence, both from formal studies and anecdotal observations, that cannabis may truly be helpful for people with MS. Pain, sleep deprivation, emotional changes like anxiety and depression and spasticity all improve with weed. Cannabis is already providing relief to patients in 15 countries via prescription, but unfortunately, patients in the U.S. do not have this choice. Until the FDA gets on board, cannabis may be an alternative to explore for some Americans.

Pain

If you didn't read the chapter before this on pot and painkillers, I'll topline it here. Cannabis helps with multiple types of pain: neuropathic (burning), mechanical (aching) and inflammatory (acute, sharp). THC, in concert with the full range of cannabinoids, is a safe and, for many, effective treatment option for all kinds of pain. On its own or as a boost to opioids, the THC in weed can make you less painfully aware of what hurts. CBD, with its anti-inflammatory benefits, can soothe and bring ease to the body.

For every condition listed here that is accompanied by chronic pain; for every person whose body is facing a lot more aches and pains; for every being that suffers from something—cannabis can be a path to relief. Naturally, safely and without risk of long-term effects. Side effects are generally manageable, and minimized or eliminated when the right weed is matched with the right person. Don't count on the person behind the counter to know what will work for you. We'll get into this later, but we each have our own unique chemistry and connection with cannabis.

And for those who "just say no" to opioids, marijuana might just be a "yes." Or at the very least, a "maybe." With such strong evidence to its benefits and very few red flags, cannabis deserves serious consideration. It is proving to be a viable alternative for prescription painkillers and a pathway from dependence and addiction for those of us with chronic pain.

Parkinson's Disease

Another insidious disease, Parkinson's is a degenerative disorder of the nervous system, which causes the motor system to fail over time. Michael J. Fox and Katherine Hepburn are two of the most well-known sufferers. Tremors and shaking, muscle rigidity and spasms are the worst of the symptoms, which start subtle and get progressively worse until full loss of control over bodily movement. There is no cure, and the cause is unknown. Unfortunately, by the time symptoms arrive, the bulk of the damage is done.

The root cause of Parkinson's is the death of dopamine, a chemical that sends messages to the part of the brain that controls movement and coordination. (What causes the death of these neurotransmitter cells is still unknown.) Without dopamine in the system, motor skills start to shut down. Slowly.

While research is, of course, limited, there is growing evidence that cannabis may provide tremor relief and even more miraculous: some research is showing that its neuroprotective qualities may even slow the progression of the disease. We know there is a large concentration of endocannabinoid receptors in the region of the brain responsible for mobility; and that the endocannabinoid system (ECS) is affected when dopamine cells die. It looks like weed works with our ECS to modulate the release of dopamine and may even improve motor impairment. Treatment may lie within our own ECS! It's not crazy to think that cannabis could have positive results; cannabinoid receptors hang out in great numbers in the area important to Parkinson's disease. So, when the cannabinoids in cannabis go to the brain, they also go to where Parkinson's hangs out and does its damage.

When it comes to treating Parkinson's, patients don't have a lot of options. Medical marijuana is helping many cope with tremors and side effects from medication, which can be debilitating in and of themselves. And stories and dramatic videos are cropping up with increasing frequency about patients who find (nearly) complete (albeit temporary) relief from consuming cannabis, who stop shaking and can talk while under the effect of this drug with "zero medicinal value."

Post Traumatic Stress Disorder (PTSD)

Veterans with PTSD are on the front lines of the war on weed and many are fighting hard to make marijuana available; ideally, this time they'll come out on the winning side. Twenty-two veterans a day are lost to suicide; you can be pretty sure PTSD is part of the mix.

Trauma comes from many sources, not just combat; and for any man or woman suffering from PTSD, it's very real and very debilitating, causing things like severe panic attacks and haunting nightmares. People with PTSD get flashbacks, sometimes triggered by something as simple as a sound or scent. Anger, outbursts, social avoidance, irritability, insomnia, depression and anxiety often accompany the trauma throughout life.

Like with clinical depression and anxiety, a brain with PTSD is sending out way too much stress hormones and adrenaline, and is lacking in anandamide (the bliss molecule, the one that THC replicates... remember from earlier?) The result? Fear, reliving bad memories and chronic anxiety. THC, CBD and the other cannabinoids signal the brain to deactivate traumatic memories.

Patients with PTSD are often prescribed a cocktail of pharmaceutical drugs that can include antidepressants, anti-anxiety drugs, sleeping pills, and even antipsychotics. Few drugs work; most don't. Most have some pretty awful side effects. But many patients, and far more than the record will show, are using weed to treat their symptoms. While the evidence accumulates, astounding numbers of people are taking matters into their own hands (or lungs, in this case). One study found patients who smoked pot experienced a 75% reduction in symptoms.

The FDA has finally approved clinical trials for using cannabis to treat PTSD and the VA just approved medical marijuana for our vets; but we're still a ways off from any substantive progress in officially having cannabis-based drugs to treat PTSD. But even without the Fed's blessing, it's only a matter of time before the medical community and government begins to understand and accept the fact that weed is a simple, safe and effective treatment for PTSD and a (better) alternative to pharmaceuticals. It has the power to control the symptoms of PTSD and help people lead normal, productive lives. Not quite the havoc on lives weed supposedly wreaks!

Weight Management

Weed can play a dual role with your appetite and weight, regulating not just whether you want to eat (or not), but potentially blood sugar as well. If you recall, those of us who consume cannabis tend to have a healthier body weight than our non-toking brethren.

Weed does have a legendary reputation for stimulating the appetite. The munchies are a very good "side effect" for people suffering through cancer treatment and chronic, debilitating diseases.

But on the flip side, pot also seems to help people slim down and maintain a healthy body weight. Researchers have found that despite consuming more calories overall, marijuana users have smaller waists, lower body mass indexes and better cholesterol numbers than those who pass on grass. And while scientists are still figuring it out, they think weed helps regulate the production of insulin and helps efficiently manage calories. Those who toke up have less incidences of diabetes. Perhaps a joint a day keeps the doctor away…. How 'bout them apples?

—

Cannabis is inherently polypharmaceutical, which means it can take on multiple roles and even replace multiple medications. For most, cannabis is safe and well-tolerated, and carries fewer risks of adverse drug interactions than many other commonly prescribed drugs. As such, cannabis can not only reduce the amount or dosage needed for a given prescription, it can also reduce the mixing of multiple medications with risk of adverse interactions. Think about it: why take six (or more) prescriptions, all of which could interact with each other, when you can take just one medicine?

5 PRESCRIPTIONS THAT COULD BE REPLACED BY WEED

1. Painkillers

2. Benzos/anti-anxiety meds

3. Stimulants

4. Sleeping pills

5. Anti-depressants

By the way, a recent survey just did a deep dive into CBD and its usage and effectiveness; and guess what? Nearly half the people who use CBD stop taking traditional medicine. And in a break with the stereotype of the male cannabis consumer, women are more likely than men to use CBD. The most common reasons to use CBD? To treat Insomnia, depression, anxiety and joint pain.

MARIJUANA, MENSTRUATION & MENOPAUSE

We may not yet know exactly why and how, but we have known for hundreds of years that cannabis can ease menstrual and menopausal symptoms. Remember our lesson on the ECS? It plays a critical role in maintaining homeostasis and regulating functions like body temperature, sleep, mood, metabolism and reproductive cycles. Endocannabinoid and estrogen levels are closely linked, and can have big impact on women's health—estrogen levels peak during ovulation (making us more sensitive to THC, be aware!), and then are reduced as we move into menopause.

For women suffering from PMS, cramps and other unpleasant period symptoms, cannabis can provide an incredibly effective path for self care. Its pain-relieving, muscle-relaxing effects can ease cramping and discomfort, back and belly pain, gastrointestinal issues, breast tenderness and even headaches. And marijuana's mood-elevating properties and ability to promote a sense of positivity and well-being can help with the emotional ups and downs that come with hormonal shifts.

As estrogen is reduced in the body, so are endocannabinoids, which may be responsible for those not-so-pleasant symptoms associated with menopause: hot flashes, mood issues and bone loss. For women in the "hot zone" of menopause (and particularly for those of us who cannot take traditional estrogen replacement therapy (ERT) treatment), marijuana can be a powerful tool for natural relief: cannabis can boost serotonin signaling and lower body temperature, which can reduce hot flashes, stress, anxiety and depression. Cannabinoids have been found to stimulate bone growth and may stave off osteoporosis. Sleep improves. So does sex drive and responsiveness. And, contrary to its association with the munchies, cannabis many actually help with weight management and insulin sensitivity.

Simply put, cannabis is a safe and viable treatment for a wide range of issues that come with having lady parts.

What About Interactions With Other Medications?

Chemical compounds interact with other chemical compounds. For example, there are 82 drug interactions with caffeine. Even grapefruit interacts with some drugs. When it comes to cannabis, most potential interactions are relatively mild.

In fact, some drugs seem to work together with cannabis favorably, increasing the effectiveness or potency. As with painkillers, cannabis can be synergistic and create an effect greater than the sum of the parts. Or, with other meds, it can simply be additive.

It's important to remember that cannabis is not a single drug; it's a complex plant comprised of numerous compounds. Cannabinoid and terpene profiles vary from strain to strain, and so their effects and potential interactions, both good and bad, can vary as well.

There is minimal clinical research around cannabis and interactions. Reports of negative interactions are few, and as I frequently reiterate, take it 'low and slow.' A little bit of cannabis isn't going to put you at risk or do long term damage. Even if the interaction is potentially beneficial, you'll want to work with your doctor(s) and monitor your blood work in case you need to adjust your medication's dosage.

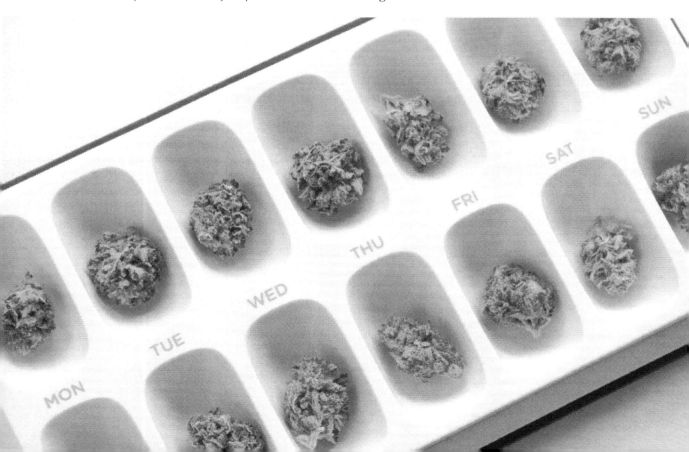

If you or a loved one is taking prescriptions, here are a few considerations to discuss with your physician if your medication falls into one of these categories:

Blood sugar: While direct data correlating cannabinoids to blood sugar levels is not yet available, there is increasing evidence that cannabis lowers insulin resistance and improves control over blood sugar (and therefore may help combat obesity). If you are on medication, glucose levels could be lowered and should be monitored appropriately.

Blood pressure: Because THC activates both CB1 and CB2 receptors, it can lower blood pressure. While reports of adverse events are relatively rare, cannabis may compound effects of blood-pressure meds.

Blood thinners: Both THC and CBD may increase the duration of action and effect for drugs like warfarin used for blood thinning by possibly slowing down their breakdown/metabolism. Lower doses of blood thinners may be indicated to reduce risk of bleeding.

Sedatives: Cannabinoids like CBD and THC, as well as terpenes like myrcene and linalool, can produce sedative effects. Unlike alcohol, which can be deadly, cannabis doesn't elevate blood levels or amplify the effects of sedatives. That said, the effect is additive—you may get even more tired and drowsy—and so they should be used with caution together.

Depending on what, how much, how often and in what format you consume cannabis, it's possible that you will have side effects commonly associated with being high. Dizziness, dry mouth, loss of balance and impaired memory/cognition are all potential effects from weed. In the next section, we'll get into how to consume responsibly and manage your high (or lack thereof) to have the best experience possible, but any and all of these are possible effects.

For people with anxiety or mania, the wrong weed can exacerbate symptoms and so introducing cannabis should be done with care. Most definitely avoid a high-THC strain or product and remember that CBD helps mitigate anxiety. I will continue to beat the drum of "go low and slow." In doing so, any potential uncomfortable side effects will be limited and short-lived. The only real safety issue, and legitimately so for someone older and anyone driving, is loss of balance and dizziness. The weed won't do any harm, but a fall most certainly could.

Marijuana Doesn't Have to Be Medical to be Therapeutic

There's no doubt cannabis can play a significant role in helping people find legitimate relief and healing from illness, disease and chronic conditions. It's a compelling reason to consider cannabis as a replacement or supplement to many medications; and just might be the most versatile, holistic tool available to physicians throughout the ages and well into the future.

With all the excitement and focus on medical marijuana, it's easy to brush off recreational use and leave that to the stoners. But wouldn't you agree that hearing music can lift your spirits? Or enjoying a meal with friends? Watching the sun rise or set? Well, it's all better on weed! They say laughter is the best medicine—so what's wrong with getting the giggles and laughing at the dog?

> **"**The illegality of cannabis is outrageous, an impediment to full utilization of a drug which helps produce the serenity and insight, sensitivity and fellowship so desperately needed in this increasingly mad and dangerous world.**"**

CARL SAGAN
American Astronomer and Scientist

Marijuana amplifies sensual pleasures: sight, smell, touch, sound and taste are all elevated when THC mimics or modulates chemicals like dopamine and serotonin that our bodies naturally produce. Colors are brighter, food tastes better, things are funnier. It can produce waves of creativity, moments of inspiration and cohesive thinking and bright ideas. Weed induces feelings of well-being and happiness. Inspires wonder and awe. It helps people relax and unwind, get a restful night's sleep, connect with themselves and each other, find inspiration, feel joy and stay present. Stress is by far one of our society's most insidious and pervasive issues—less of it can only be a good thing, don't you think?

These benefits are more healing to humans than we tend to think; don't underestimate the power of gratitude, contentment, presence and love...all of which can be brought forward mindfully and responsibly with weed by the vast majority of people.

The Plant That Can Heal the World

If cannabis was discovered in the middle of the jungle today, it would make headlines worldwide as a miracle drug and game-changing industrial crop. The sad thing is that it was discovered thousands of years ago, recognized and appreciated for its value, and then got caught up in politics, big money, racism, xenophobia and fear. For nearly 100 years, the plant has been shoved in a dark, dank closet and the world has been deprived of its potential and its value.

This plant has application at an industrial level through agricultural hemp and big medicine. It's renewable and versatile, and can help create hundreds of thousands of products, from food to fuel, composite materials to medicine. (Big Pharma may not be happy about all the ways weed can help people wean off pharmaceuticals, but you can rest assured they will not lose out on the multi-billion dollar market opportunity that will open up once the government gets synched up with its citizens, scientists and health professionals). Cannabis can help communities, individuals, society, pets and the planet in ways bigger and more powerful than we can possibly imagine.

We are making progress, but people are still being fed painkillers and prescriptions in record numbers. Pot has potential to be a real solution to the opioid crisis, so much so the government is being sued for legalization. Alcohol and tobacco are proven to be deadly and harmful, yet are accepted as societal norms and marketable, lightly-regulated businesses. Too many people are still being locked up and facing asset forfeiture.

Weed works. Not for everyone and not for everything, but it does have proven capacity to do great things for people. This is not "crazy liberal talk." Once you get past any misguided perceptions about marijuana's supposed dangers, the rest is just common sense. Used intentionally and with care, cannabis can be a tool for people to reconnect with themselves and their bodies, as well as their loved ones and the world around them.

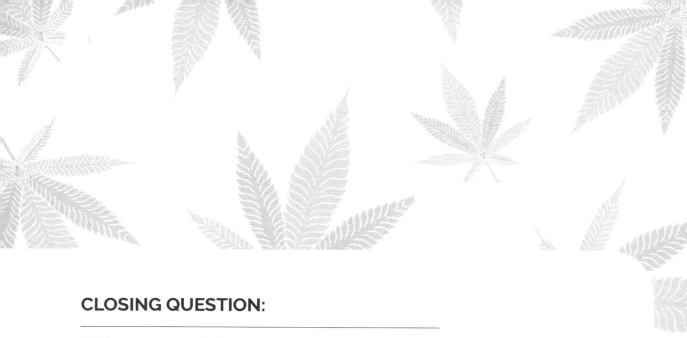

What conditions can't cannabis treat?

We're still figuring out the many ways weed can help the multitudes suffering in so many ways. Some conditions are clearly at the head of the pack in terms of what we know and how we're targeting cannabinoid therapies. Others will come to the front as new insights and data are brought forward. But generally speaking, if it's connected to your ECS, there's a good chance cannabis can help your condition.

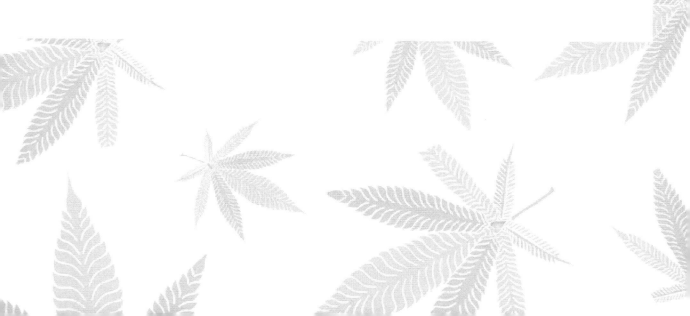

CATCHING UP: MEET THE NEW WEED, (NOT THE) SAME AS THE OLD WEED

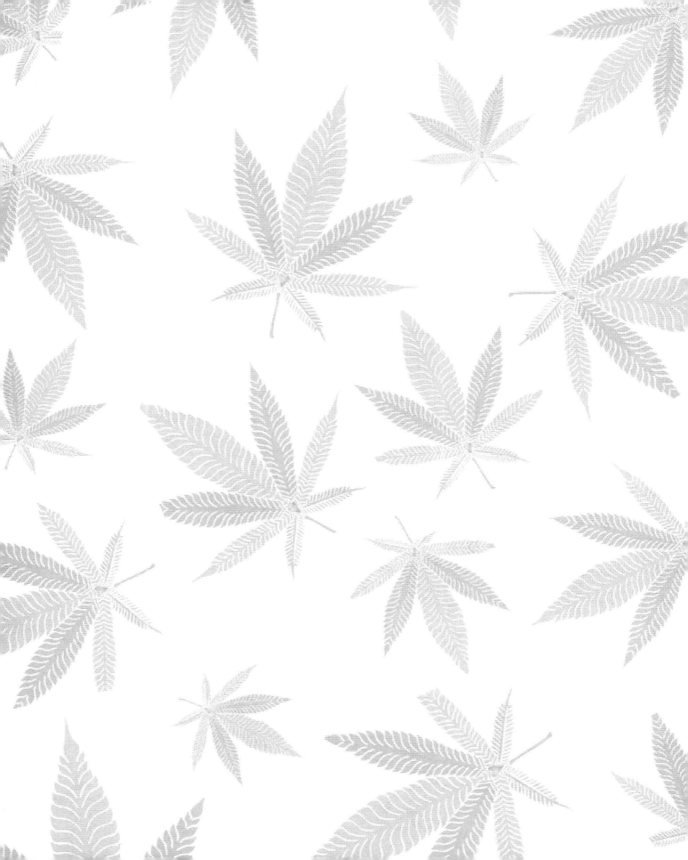

11 | LET'S START WITH THE LINGO

I hope I've done my job as a communicator and gotten you comfortable with the fact that cannabis is proven to provide relief and healing to many. But comfortable with the safety and efficacy of cannabis and comfortable with choosing and consuming it are very different, so let's focus on more practical applications of your knowledge, okay?

The world of weed has a language all its own. In some ways it was created as code to let stoners communicate with each other when parents, teachers, police officers or others who "aren't cool" are around. In others, it's just part of our cultural fabric and reflects the stoner subculture and the wild creativity that emerges from the haze of smoke.

There are countless terms for cannabis itself; 1,200 and growing at last count. And if you want to get high? Well, you might get elevated, blazed, baked or lit while smoking a fatty or doobie (or a 'J') with your buds. Your budtender will set you up for your next sesh. Just make sure to tell him or her that you don't want to get high if that's not your jam. You don't need to worry about a contact high unless you're hotboxing in a car or other confined space.

Keep reading and you'll learn how to avoid couchlock, prepare for cottonmouth and be ready in case you end up with a creeper and unexpectedly find yourself higher than you want to be. (Hint: have some CBD on hand.) You'll know to always pass the joint to the left, and to not bogart it when it does come to you. It's puff, puff, pass…not puff, puff, pause to reflect. If you're the last one standing when the bowl is cashed, it's time to pack a new one; but at least you get first-hit privileges.

The world of weed has a broad and highly descriptive vocabulary, and it grows daily. For those of us who speak the language regularly, we sling a lot of lingo around; so here's a rundown of some of the most common terms and a quick language lesson.

CANNABIS CAN ALSO BE CALLED:

Marijuana

Weed

Pot

Ganja

Herb

Bud

Mary Jane

Dank

Grass

Chronic

Reefer

Dope

Wacky Tabacky*

The Devil's Lawn Clippings

420

*Don't actually try to use this term with anyone under the age of 40; you will likely get a blank stare or an eye roll.

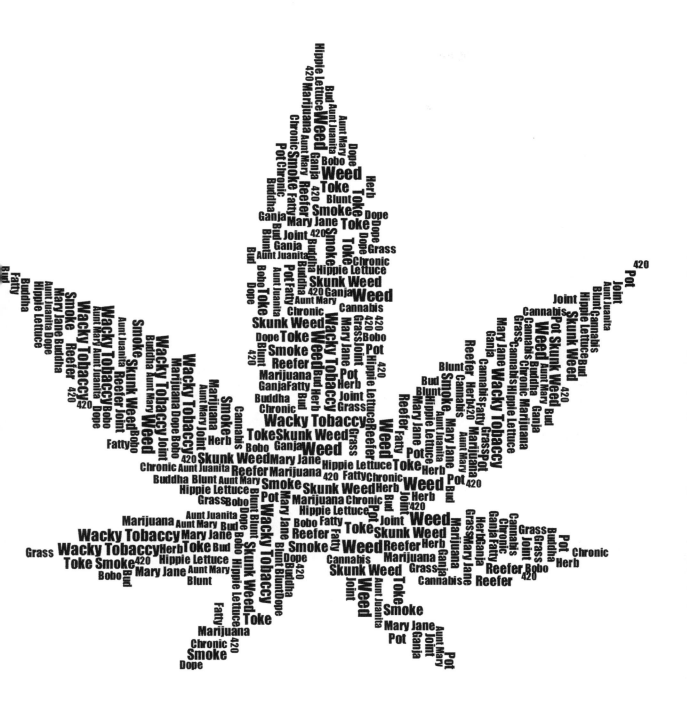

What's the Deal with 420?

"420" may be one of the most ubiquitous slang terms for weed. Whether as reference for pot itself, the act of consuming it or an identifier that you indeed "are cool" (420-friendly), it's shorthand term that signals something weed-related in both stoner and mass culture. But what do these three little numbers mean? Where did this universal code for weed come from?

Well, it seems a group of five friends in California known as the Waldos—by virtue of their chosen hang-out spot, a wall outside the school—coined the term in 1971. Every afternoon at 4:20 they'd meet to go on a hunt for a small crop of abandoned marijuana plants. 420 became their codeword for the daily search; they never found the mystery crop but continued to use the term for anything marijuana-related. Some in the Waldos were connected to and hung out with the Grateful Dead, and 420 got picked up as lingo for weed within the Dead's subculture and, from there, it spread to the rest of the world. The term 420 went viral before going viral was a thing.

WAYS TO TALK ABOUT WEED

You pack a bowl (in a pipe or bong) and take a hit, toking up until the bowl or joint is cashed. When it's done, either clean and re-pack the bowl or roll yourself a new joint.

You can medicate with marijuana. Or, you can also get super baked on some dank weed. You can also get elevated with fine artisanal cannabis from a local grower.

People with chronic conditions often wake and bake, getting started early in the day to manage symptoms and minimize medications.

People get together or go outside for a sesh; hopefully no one bogarts the joint. The rule of thumb is "puff, puff, pass." (and always to the left).

If you get cottonmouth or the munchies from weed, as long as you avoid couchlock you can quench your thirst or hunger with a quick trip to the kitchen. Or Taco Bell, since it's pretty much always open.

Once you've finished your sesh, put away your stash somewhere secure and safe from animals or kids. Even if it's not deadly, cannabis should only be consumed by consenting adults.

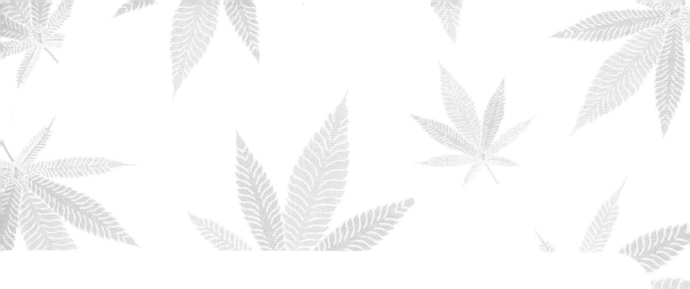

CLOSING QUESTION:

Why are there so many euphemisms and ways to talk about weed?

Marijuana has been kept underground for so long that it has developed a unique and far-reaching subculture. People who consumed had to create a new language to communicate with each other, which has flourished and evolved as the audience has grown along with the culture. I wonder what new terms and language will come out of this new consumer influx into the cannabis culture?

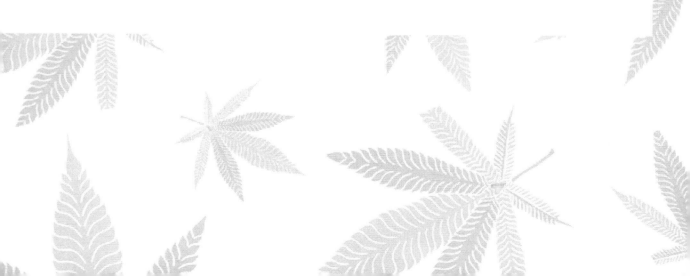

12 | SO MANY STRAINS, SO LITTLE STANDARDIZATION

Even if you've toked up here and there over the years, if you're not an active cannabis consumer, chances are you have little to no familiarity with the difference between an indica or a sativa; and there's a good chance you probably don't even know what those words even mean. If so, not to worry; we'll get there in just a bit. (By the way, until recently Willie Nelson didn't even know the difference between a sativa and an indica, and he's pretty much the poster child of potheads!)

So here's the thing: Yes, strains are categorized as sativas, indicas or hybrids—but the reality of what's behind any given strain name and designation isn't all that real. Conventional wisdom and the foundational principles of strains and the effects they deliver are proving to be pretty far off the mark. It ends up the way the community names its plants and the way we're coached to choose our cannabis is all messed up.

Weed's Family Tree—
Turns Out It's Not What We Thought

Let's go back to the roots of cannabis for a moment, because that is the source of the original categorization. Marijuana originated in South and Central Asia, evolving into two distinct species to accommodate different environments and humidity regimes. Sativa has thin, lanky stems and long leaves to respirate more efficiently and prosper in high humidity; short, squat indicas evolved to deal with hot, dry conditions. The original strains of indica developed in the dry foothills of the Himalayas, while pure sativas evolved in humid low-lands and river valleys. "Pure" varieties from the original sources are called landrace strains.

Weed's family tree starts with these landrace strains, with everything branching off from there. We've built a classification system based on it and use it to guide how strains are named and categorized. It's the closest thing to standardization at the moment. By today's standards, I'd be able to trace the lineage of my Sour Diesel to the strains: Original Diesel and DNL. I should also be able to predict its effects based on this genetic profile.

But here's the thing; as plants have been bred and cross-bred, the genetics have intermingled and most of what we have here in the U.S. is one indica-sativa hybrid or another. We're starting to conduct genetic testing on cannabis and the data coming back doesn't often support the indica/sativa divide. Strains considered sativas are coming back as being genetically almost identical to some indicas. The labels don't synch up with the genetics.

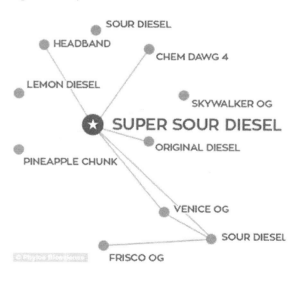

It goes beyond genetics—growing conditions make a difference, creating plants with new traits and unique cannabinoid profiles, which as I hope you recall, is really what is important in evaluating and categorizing cannabis.

We're Doing It All Wrong: Why Labels Don't Matter

Remember earlier I referenced we are all unique—a sativa for me could have a different effect than it will on you; not just based on our individual endocannabinoid systems and other factors, but also because every strain has its own cannabinoid profile. And, as we just covered, genetic variability and growing conditions could produce plants of the same strain with varying profiles and effects. A Sour Diesel may not actually be a Sour Diesel, or may not end up feeling like the Sour D I've come to know and love. (And for medical patients, this could be important.)

We are told to look for a sativa if we want a head-high or energy, and that an indica will give us couchlock. While sativa and indica labels are valid for describing the physical characteristics of the strain, they aren't as reliable to use as a predictor of their effects and how you're going to feel. What can give you a reliable sense of what to expect? Two things: THC and terpenes.

Both indicas and sativas contain the full complement of cannabinoids and terpenes—but it's the THC which produces a euphoric, uplifting sensation when consumed. The higher the concentration of THC, the higher you will get. It's pretty straightforward on that front.

> The twist in the plot comes with terpenes (remember them?) and in particular, with myrcene. If you'll recall, terpenes are what bring flavor and aroma to weed (and other plants and foods), and are key to shaping the effects we feel from one strain to another. Indicas, as it turns out, tend to be especially heavy in myrcene, which flips the switch from a euphoric, energetic high (which sounds a lot like how a sativa is described) to couchlock. The higher the levels of myrcene, the more sedative and stony the effects will be.

All this said, the industry generally still goes by the indica/sativa designation as the driver behind a strain or product's label. Budtenders and the vast majority of people still use it as a way to talk about and recommend products. And actual labeling with test results and terpene profiles is still pretty uncommon, so knowing the percentage of myrcene is pretty much impossible unless you have access to an outside testing lab or one at home. Until the market catches up, you'll still need to know the basic foundation for categorizing weed.

Before long, we won't even be using sativa or indica as the basis for which strain to choose—the cannabinoid profile and desired effects will be the decision factors between one strain or product and another. Many brands have already bypassed this construct and created products designed to deliver a mood or an effect. Variations on "Sleep," "Bliss," "Relax," "Focus," "Pain" and other packaged experiences are aiming to be more consumer-friendly and becoming more readily available in marijuana markets across the country, and will certainly continue to be the norm.

But until then and to get you started, these broad strokes of how sativas, indicas and hybrids work should give you a foundation for deciding what kind of product or strain to try. And it can help you be confident in making the right choice even if you have no idea if Alaskan Thunderfuck (yes, a real strain) will get you riled up or zonked out (as a sativa-dominant strain, riled up is most likely).

For now, just remember: a sativa will get you high; an indica will get you stoned.

THE ABCS OF WEED ARE AS EASY AS 1-2-3

Sativa: Generally a more energetic and uplifting effect, giving a cerebral "head high." Artists, writers and musicians appreciate sativas for sparking creativity and inspiration. For people with nausea, sativas are known to both battle the nausea and be an appetite stimulator. As a rule of thumb, good for the daytime. But, hit it too much or use high-THC strain, and you might find yourself spacey or with a racy brain.

Indica: More of a "body high," indicas lean toward relaxation and a heavier, stoned feeling—think of it as "in da couch." Great for helping with pain management and a better night's rest, and finding a calm, serene center inside yourself. With its body melt effects, too much indica can lead to couchlock and leave you with little to zero motivation. Many pot smokers partake of their indica in the evening. When you think of the stoner stereotype, too much indica is probably the culprit.

Hybrid: To state the obvious, a hybrid is some ratio of sativa-to-indica within the strain. 80/20, 70/30, 50/50 and along those lines—the variations are endless. Most strains are a hybrid, even if a heavily-leaning one, to bring forward the best qualities of both sativa and indica. Once you're familiar with how different strains work for you, you can start fine tuning your experience based on a strain's profile.

What's in a Name?

If you have any familiarity with weed over the years, you've likely heard of some of the more popular strains as they've come and gone over time. From Acapulco Gold and Maui Wowie to Green Crack and Gorilla Glue, strain names are prolific (8,000+ and growing), oftentimes wildly creative (my fellow branders, take note) and can vary wildly in regional popularity and availability.

Strain names range from whimsical to seriously profound. Some of the most famous ones originated from the history of their evolution. Many are named by their growers (many of whom were probably high for the naming session). Others are the products of urban mythology. A few are just plain marketing hype, working hard to capture your attention when it's time to buy.

There's no rhyme or reason to the naming system for marijuana strains, which is why it's so important to understand indicas and sativas and the various effects they deliver. I'll give you some guidance around how to pick the right strain in the next section, so you're not completely on your own!

For those serious about their weed, a strain's lineage gives a complex and rich picture of what kind of experience it can be expected to deliver. Ask a grower or budtender about a strain and its origins and you'll get a detailed family tree of how it's a cross between this strain and that, or a clone of an original award-winning strain. (Wait until that expands into cannabinoid and terpene profiles!)

STRAIN NAME OR BAND NAME?

Test your strain savvy.

1. Golden Goat
2. Hoobastank
3. Trainwreck
4. Chocolope
5. Purple Urkle
6. Chumbawamba
7. Jerry Garcia
8. The Mr. T Experience
9. Blue Dream
10. Afgooey
11. Mojo Nixon
12. Alaskan Thunderfuck
13. Albino Rhino
14. Hog's Breath
15. Dirty Sanchez

Answer Key:
Strain Name: 1, 3, 4, 5, 7 (gotcha!), 9, 10, 12 (softball), 14
Band Name: 2, 6, 8, 11, 13, 15

Some strains are bred for the highest THC possible; others are now being grown to meet specific cannabinoid profiles with targeted therapeutic benefits. Until there is regulation at a national level and industry standards, the best bet is to approach weed on a spectrum of sativa-ness and indica-ness and use THC, CBD and terpene profiles as the best indicators of what that strain should deliver.

TWO FOUR-LETTERED WORDS TO REMEMBER: HAZE & KUSH

Many of the most popular strains on the market come from Kush or Haze lineage, and you'll see them quite often tacked on to the end of their names. Both are known for their euphoric and happy feeling, but Hazes are more energetic and Kushes more sedative. Much like sativas and indicas, how about that? If you read "Kush" or "Haze" behind a strain, here's what you'll likely taste, smell and see:

Kush: indica dominant, tend to have a sweet and sour odor, offering smooth and complex flavors filled with notes of flowers, grape, citrus, diesel and earth. Kush varieties are brightly colored, with deep green and rich purples. Kushes are typically heavier indica varieties, providing significant body sedation and pain relief.

Haze: sativa dominant, have fresh odors and taste "brighter" with earthy-sweet citrus profiles. Buds are lighter green with lots of hairy bright orange pistils covering the outside of the flower. Among sativas, Hazes are heavy-hitting with potent cerebral and social head highs accompanied by a body brightness.

Terroir, Varietals and Regions: How Weed is Like Wine

There are 6,000 grape varietals, each with a distinct flavor, aroma and appearance. We have around 8,000 strains of marijuana, all with unique cannabinoid profiles and combinations of potency, smell and taste. In terms of its production and the overall construct, weed is a lot like wine.

We have a fundamental categorization of red/white/rose and indica/sativa/hybrid. There are different regions like the Emerald Triangle in California or Mexico which are known for the cannabis they produce, like Napa Valley in California or France for wine. People prefer specific types of wine, much like they do strains—and mix it up based on the desired experience. And for those who get into it, they'll have specific wine producers on their roster of favorites, as some cannabis enthusiasts will have with growers.

Growing weed isn't all that different from grapes, though I'm sure there are vast differences if you talk to a vintner and grower. (Weed can be grown indoors or out, in a greenhouse, under the sun or produced with mass efficiency inside warehouses.) But whether weed or wine, those who grow it will pride themselves on their unique cultivation processes, environment (terroir if the plants are grown in soil) and final product. Although weed does in fact grow like a weed, it requires a lot of work to grow organically, efficiently and on a commercial scale.

It won't be too long before regions known for their terroir and varietals become travel destinations for weekend weed-tastings and getaways. Oregon and California are already known for both their wine and weed; and you can rest assured tourist boards and startups are working on business plans right now to cater to a whole new set of clientele. As interest in production takes root like it does for wines, people will want to see where their favorite strain is grown, sesh with the head grower and get to know the people and the process behind the pot they have grown to love and appreciate.

WEED IS TO WINE...	
Garden (aka "Grow")	Vineyard
Strain	Varietal
THC/CBD/Cannabinonid Profile	Alcohol Percentage
Dispensary	Wine Shop
Terpenes	Tannins

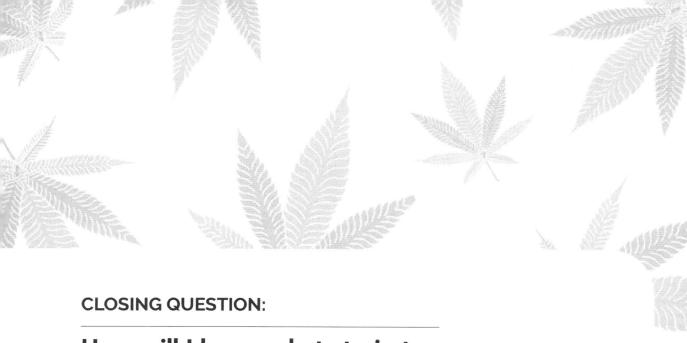

CLOSING QUESTION:

How will I know what strain to choose when the time comes?

It depends on a variety of factors. While it's no longer just about indica or sativa, they are still the foundation for how strains and products are classified. Start with an idea of where you want to be on the spectrum from sedated to energetic. From there, use terpenes and THC/CBD ratios to shape the direction of where you want to go with your weed.

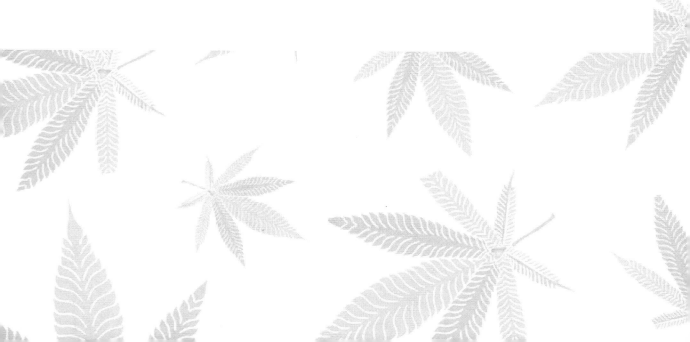

13 | DIFFERENT TOKES FOR DIFFERENT FOLKS

Weed can be consumed as flower, the dried plant material that is typically associated with what people think about marijuana. (Also referred to as bud, ganja or grass, and hopefully not ditchweed!) Flower, in turn, can be processed into concentrates or extracts, which basically remove the plant material and leave behind the essential materials and compounds for consumption in a variety of ways. Concentrates can be found in the form of oils, waxes, shatter (like hard candy, but far less tasty) and other extracted products, for ingestion through a variety of methods from smoking to sublingual absorption. We'll break it all down in the next chapter—I won't leave you hanging!

If you haven't set foot in a dispensary yet, you'll be surprised (and likely, overwhelmed) by the number of options you have to consume cannabis. As we covered earlier, you don't have to smoke a joint or make a pipe out of an apple to enjoy weed (but I'll show you how in the next section, in case you want to!) In fact, the fastest growing forms of consumption involve no combustion at all. By the way, you don't even have to inhale if you don't want.

Let me give you a run-through of the various ways you can take cannabis into your body:

Via Your Lungs

Smoking

Still the most popular form with the majority of people, weed can be rolled into joints or packed into bowls within hand pipes or bongs. You can also enjoy a blunt (a joint wrapped in cigar paper) or a spliff (a mix of weed and tobacco) if you're so inclined. Glass pipes can be beautiful, practical and efficient, ranging from functional to an art piece. Bongs use water to filter the smoke, making for a cooler, smoother hit. By the way, bongwater tastes and smells awful, so keeping it clean is pretty important if you don't want a mouthful of foul backsplash. Like with pipes, bongs can vary in their beauty and cost. Both glass pipes and bongs can also be fragile, so if you're like me and can't have nice things, don't buy the prettiest pipe or most beautiful bong you find until you see how you handle things... literally and figuratively.

These forms of consumption involve burning of the plant material through direct flame. For some, concerns over releasing toxic chemicals from the combustion itself or perhaps the harshness of hot smoke in the lungs is a deterrent. Have no fear; there is a better way to inhale!

Vaporizing

Many people confuse smoking with vaping—don't make that mistake. They are not the same thing. Vaporizers heat marijuana at temperatures high enough to release the cannabinoids and terpenes, but low enough to avoid combustion from burning the marijuana with a flame. With vaping, you still inhale (but don't hold—we'll get into the how-tos in the next section), but what you're getting is a lungful of vapor that has almost no residual smell and is cooler than smoke.

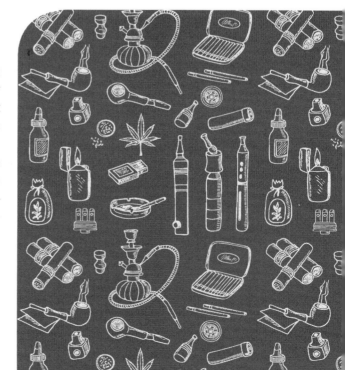

You can vaporize either flower or concentrate, using either a desktop device or a hand-held vape pen. The market is flooded with vaporizers of every size, shape, style and price point, from disposable to durable. We'll get more into the different tools in the next section, but vaping can be a highly efficient and effective way to get whatever benefits you're seeking from weed and give you a cleaner, more flavorful experience. And its discretion can't be beat—with virtually no odor and devices that are indistinguishable from common items like pens, lipstick or electronic cigarettes, vaping is a versatile option for just about anyone.

Vaping is the fastest growing form of consumption, largely because of its discretion, ease and manageability of the experience. Most doctors prefer vaporizing for their medical marijuana patients. It's by far the easiest entry into consumption, as the effects are both immediate and relatively short-lived. If the experience isn't working, it's easy enough to change it up and look for the right product or strain in another sesh (remember, sesh = consumption session).

Dabbing

Not for the novice, dabbing is a relatively new form of consumption available on the market. (It's been around for a decade or so, but is becoming more popular as access to cannabis concentrates continues to expand.) It is the hottest trend in weed today, particularly with Millennials. The term comes from placing a "dab" of concentrate on a superheated piece of metal called a nail. When the dab hits the heat, it vaporizes and releases all those good cannabinoids within the extract.

The media trots out images of 20-somethings taking huge dabs off elaborate paraphernalia ("dab rigs") and warn people about this new craze. Dabbing can be a high-intensity way to get high, but it can also be done sensibly, intentionally and safely. We are using concentrated cannabis here, so getting too high is entirely too possible without care and caution. I've seen people take way too much and get lightheaded, dizzy and even faint—but I've also seen people enjoy a super tasty hit delivered by a responsible server in concert with an elegant dinner event. We'll get more into how to consume sensibly in the next section, but coming out of the gate, this is not where a "canna-newb" should start exploring cannabis unless you're being guided by a "canna-professional."

Dabbing can be a highly sophisticated and nuanced experience, but it can also be the equivalent of shotgunning a beer (or, more like it, a bottle of liquor.) Heating the nail is done either through a butane torch (thus making dabbing seem like doing crack) or through an electronic nail which is digitally controlled. At super high temperatures, dabbing can get you super high (again, reinforcing the crack reference.) But lower temperatures are where the magic happens, heating the concentrate to whatever level releases the flavors and aromas from those tasty terpenes, as well as the various cannabinoids hanging out in the concentrates. For the "cannaseur," it's like being able to enjoy all the nuances found in a good wine (or tea, if wine isn't your thing)! And for the patient, it provides a highly controllable and precise way to medicate.

Through Your Mouth

Edibles & Beverages

We've come a long way since the iconic pot brownie; it has some serious competition in the culinary space. From high-end truffles to salty snacks, root beer to your morning joe, the number of things you can medicate and put into your mouth is practically endless. If it has fat in it, you can put weed in it. Or, weed extract to be exact.

In varying formats and dosages, oral ingestion provides a longer-lasting effect than inhaling smoke or vapor and can be incredibly effective for managing pain and chronic conditions, or for staying elevated for an evening out. But how you feel on edibles is very different than you do with smoking or vaping; you should consider them different drugs, so to speak, in terms of usage. I know people who can chain-smoke joints all day long, but a single edible can take them out at the knees. This is because how your body processes THC differs depending on how you're consuming it. When you inhale marijuana, THC enters the bloodstream through your lungs, where it then has quick access to your brain (where all the psychoactivity goes down).

When weed enters the body through your mouth, it goes through the stomach and then the liver before entering your bloodstream. Your liver further breaks the THC down, converting THC from Delta-9 to 11-Hydroxy, which makes it super duper psychoactive—edibles can be five times as psychoactive as inhaled THC!

Depending on your metabolism, weight, what you ate, how much fat was in it, the consistency of the product and other factors, the effects can take anywhere from 20 minutes to two hours (and sometimes longer) to kick in—and they can last up to eight hours or longer. Done right, it's an enduring high that does what you want it to. Done wrong, it can be an enduring hell that kicks your ass (but won't actually kill you, even if you feel like you might die).

People have lost vacations to one bite too many, so when I tell you tread carefully, I do not say this lightly. The slow onset of effects has led many impatient people to believe they didn't take enough, leading to paralyzing highness and a nightmare experience. An edible high is stronger, deeper and longer than anything you can get through your lungs. As I've said again and again, until you find what works for you, the key is to "go low and slow"— 5–10 milligrams of THC is a single serving for a newbie. I'll give you plenty of guidance to prevent losing anything to weed in the next section, so keep going!

DON'T BE A MAUREEN DOWD

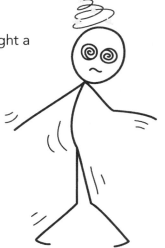

This is Maureen.

Maureen came to Colorado and bought a medicated candy bar.

Maureen should have eaten one piece (as she was told.)

Maureen ate the whole thing.

Maureen wasn't happy at all.

Don't be like Maureen.

By the way, you can't get high from eating (or juicing) raw or unactivated cannabis. Cannabinoids get activated when dissolved in lipids and heated (called decarboxylation, but we're getting ahead of ourselves; we'll get there), so they must be drawn out of the plant material with a solvent fat such as butter or oil. Cannabutter or other fat-based infusion is the foundation for cannabinated cooking, either done at home or commercially. There is also the option of infusing (or spreading) concentrated hash oil into pretty much anything, which takes edible cannabis to an entirely new level.

Drinkables are a relatively new category in the market, despite being used in India for millennia (bhang milkshakes are served at festivals and parties to this day.) Because cannabinoids need fat or another solvent (like alcohol) to release the psychoactive effects, most medicated beverages have been milk- or alcohol-based. But as cannabis concentrates become more bioavailable through technology, as well as more accessible through deregulation, hash-oil spiked sodas, juices, coffees and teas are all becoming tasty ways to medicate.

Beyond food and drink, you can ingest cannabis through pills, either formulated and packaged or made at home with hash oil in capsules. (As with edibles, the effects can take time to come on, so "low and slow" continues to be the mantra here.)

The art and science of cannabinated cooking is starting to reach new heights of inventiveness; I can't wait to see what's still to come. Imagine if Willie Wonka had weed at his disposal!

WHAT'S AN EDIBLE HIGH LIKE?

Processing through your stomach and liver creates a stronger and more pervasive physical effect. At the right dose, an edible high brings an overall sense of calmness and relaxation; it's the ultimate chill pill. If you're in pain, you'll notice you've stopped noticing it. The rest of it will depend on whether it's indica, sativa or hybrid; how much you take, how strong it is, what you're doing and how your body is feeling that day. Many people find they get productive and focused. Creative and energetic. Ideas flow. Work gets done.

Let me share a snippet from a conversation I had just the other day with my friend David:

> "I love an edible high. It's my Sunday thing! I pop a gummy and don't even notice when it starts to kick in. It doesn't hit me like a truck… it's completely mellow and I'm focused and in the zone of whatever I'm doing. I'm ridiculously productive, and I just made the best pineapple salsa I've ever made. With three kids in the house, it doesn't stink up the house and I can be discreet. We've had the conversation, but I'm still not going to consume in front of my teenagers."

On the flip side, overdosing on an edible can be a miserable experience. Too much THC flooding your system can lead to dizziness, anxiety or paranoia, a racing heart, shortness of breath, nausea, fainting and seizure-like symptoms, an inability to move and even hallucinations. Remember that despite feeling like you might be dying, you are not. You do not need to go to the ER. The only real remedy is time and relaxation (though CBD is a secret weapon, and I have a few other tips, so keep reading!)

Tinctures

Typically alcohol- or glycerin-based, tinctures contain cannabis concentrate in a solution administered via liquid drops. Taken under the tongue, tinctures absorb faster than edibles or drinkables—hitting the bloodstream as quickly as smoke or vapor. Added to food or drink, the cannabinoids will get processed more leisurely by the liver; as such, tinctures in food or beverages should be treated like an edible and waiting at least two hours before another dose is actually important, unlike waiting 20 minutes after eating before taking a swim.

Tinctures are preferred by many patients for their immediate onset (if taken under the tongue) and lasting effect. Without smoke or size, they are also discreet and portable. And, since they aren't tasty treats, you won't be tempted to overindulge.

On Your Skin

Topicals

Lotions, balms, salves and bath bombs are also ways to experience the world of cannabinoids. Applied directly to the skin, cannabis compounds go to work on sore muscles and joints, as well as on skin conditions (like psoriasis or eczema) or other issues like cuts, bruises and irritations. They can also help reduce itching and swelling, bringing inflammation down on the inside and outside of the body. From arthritis and fibromyalgia to sprains and bug bites, weed for your skin can be a very good thing.

And, we'll get into this further once we get into ways in which weed can enhance your life, but as a coming attraction (so to speak), it can also be applied topically in our nether regions for an enhanced sexual experience. Another surprising benefit!

Cannabis is loaded with vitamins, minerals and antioxidants easily absorbed through the skin with the cannabinoids. I'm sure you've seen hemp oil promoted as a key ingredient in a wide variety of bath and beauty products; perhaps you're familiar with Dr. Bronner's? Infusing these same kinds of products with marijuana in legal states can offer a broader spectrum of cannabinoids to your skin and system.

And because topicals stop short of entering the bloodstream, they aren't psychoactive and so won't get you high. I've heard some people rave about the relaxing body melt they get from taking a weed-infused bath. That could be considered high, I suppose, but in the same way you feel amazing and relaxed after a spa treatment.

Transdermals

Recent developments have brought new topical applications like controlled-release transdermal patches and roll-on lotions which can now penetrate the bloodstream. They bypass the digestive system and liver and flood your system with cannabinoids, delivering effects within minutes. Discreet, portable and for many, an effective way to medicate throughout the day.

Inside Your Body

Suppositories

Get past any potential "ew" or "tee-hee" reaction, and this may be one of the most effective cannabis delivery vehicles out there. Or in there, if you really want to get literal. By bypassing the stomach and liver, suppositories deliver THC and cannabinoids directly into the bloodstream through rectal administration. Estimates vary, but I've seen ranges of 50–80% used in terms of absorption rates. That's a lot more cannabinoids remaining to work on your endocannabinoid system. And, with zero head high and no known side effects.

Like a topical, cannabis concentrate is infused into an oil-based compound, which can then be inserted vaginally or anally to provide relief, healing or pleasure enhancement. For women suffering from menstrual issues or PCOS, cannabis-infused suppositories can maximize the muscle-relaxing and pain-relieving properties of cannabis without the psychoactive high. Fissures and hemorrhoids have been known to heal up quickly with localized "cannapplication."

And for patients suffering from disease and illness (and particularly those with digestive or urinary issues) or who can't keep food down, rectal suppositories are an incredibly effective way to deliver large doses of medicine without taking them down with a psychoactive knockout. Don't let buts about the butt be a roadblock to relief.

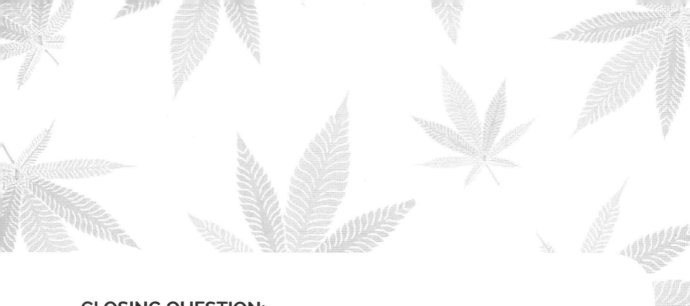

CLOSING QUESTION:

What's the best way to consume cannabis?

There is no best way. It's about what's best for you. Vaporizing or smoking provides immediate and relatively controllable effects which are short-lived, which can have both advantages and challenges. Ingestion is longer-lasting, but far harder to control and if you overdo it, you're in for a long ride. And for some people, topicals and suppositories offer good no-high options. What makes the most sense for your situation?

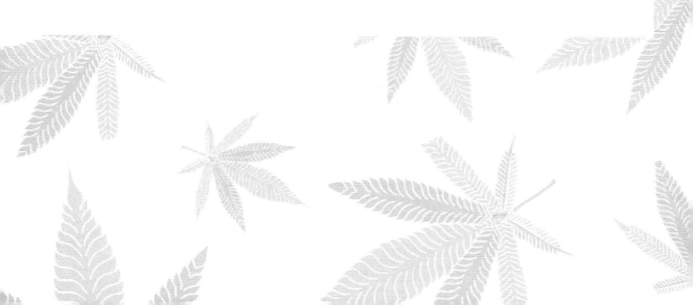

14 | A WHOLE NEW WAY TO WEED: CONCENTRATES AND EXTRACTS

Cannabis can be processed into concentrates or extracts, which strip out all the plant material and leave behind dense, sticky substances with high concentrations of cannabinoids or terpenes. THC concentrates are focused on delivering ever-higher highs, with percentages of THC reaching the upper 90s for some products. As people gain appreciation for CBD and the other cannabinoids and terpenes, and the magic they can weave, concentrates that won't take you to the limit are becoming more readily available in legal markets.

Concentrates can be found in the form of oils, waxes, shatter and other extracted products for ingestion through a variety of methods from smoking to sublingual absorption. They can be used on their own or can be added to other products to fine-tune or boost effects. As with dabbing, this can be taken to an extreme; flower dipped in hash oil, wax and kief is known as moon rocks or caviar in the weed world. (Read on for more ways to sling the lingo with confidence!) Some types of extracts are getting as high as 99.9% THC (most top out around 80%), while others rich in non-psychoactive compounds like CBD deliver an altogether "high-less" experience. For people with pain, these higher concentrations of THC can provide powerful relief in smaller doses.

Generally speaking, concentrates are portable and discreet, taking up little space and emitting little to no aroma before or after consumption. Some people like them so much they use concentrates exclusively. They can be highly effective at delivering whatever effects you're seeking, with a little bit going a long way. And for those seeking to up their cannabinoid intake, extra-strong dosing is easy and efficient.

Concentrates can be extracted through processes that use chemical solvents such as butane, CO_2 or ethanol to strip compounds from the plant, leaving behind a product jam-packed with cannabinoids. They can also be solventless through water or heat extraction.

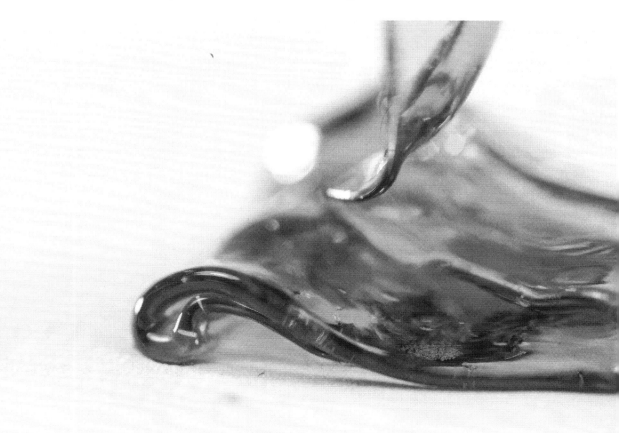

Let's break down the most common (and up-and-coming) concentrates:

Kief (pronounced "keef"): the sticky, resinous, THC-filled trichomes that cover the cannabis plant and look like pollen. It's the fine powder left at the bottom of a grinder or container. It can be smoked or vaporized, and is frequently sprinkled on flower to give it a little boost. It can be used in cooking as long as you add heat to the mix—we'll get more into this later, but most weed needs to be decarboxylized, meaning the cannabinoids are activated through heat. (And fat, but that's about absorption, not activation. It will all make sense—keep going!)

Hash: kief that's been processed and pressed into a firm substance that ranges from clay-like to a dense tar.

THC-A Crystalline: clocking in at 99.99% THC, this is the strongest hash in the world. A purified resin (white and slightly powdery, like fine small rocks) starts off benign as non-psychoactive THC-A. Activated by heat, it becomes the most potent form of consumption possible. As a pure THC concentrate, it loses the cannabinoids and terpenes that deliver the Entourage Effect I keep referencing. But, it does allow precision dosing and extremely fast relief to those who benefit from high-THC therapies.

Wax: usually made through a butane solvent extraction process, where the solvent is blasted through the plant material, removes the trichomes and then evaporates to leave behind a goopy substance that resembles—surprise!—wax.

Hash Oil: sometimes called honey oil, can be either butane or CO_2 extraction which results in a thick, viscous, resinous substance.

Shatter: goes through two butane extraction processes to create a THC-drenched substance that is smooth, glass-like and hard. Pieces are broken off and either vaporized or dabbed.

Rosin: essentially shatter without the solvents, mechanical extraction is done using heat and pressure. The result is translucent, sappy and flavorful. Fun fact: you can make rosin at home using a hair straightener! Keep reading; I'll show you how.

Cannabis Oil for Cancer (and a Whole Bunch of Other Conditions)

If you or a loved one are a medical marijuana patient, you may have heard of Rick Simpson Oil (RSO) or Phoenix Tears. In 2003 a man named Rick Simpson treated his skin cancer using a homemade cannabis oil. Medical cannabis oil is perhaps one of the most therapeutic products on the market; this whole-plant cannabis concentrate keeps every bit of cannabinoid goodness from the plant, bringing the full spectrum of healing potential into a tiny amount of a potent, sticky, dark tar-like substance.

Since then thanks to his and many others' efforts, word has spread in the cancer and medical marijuana communities about its healing potential for all kinds of conditions, including cancer, HIV/AIDS, insomnia, diabetes, depression, osteoporosis, asthma, psoriasis and more. The research isn't there, so any stories where cannabis wins over cancer are anecdotal and not evidence-based. There's no source out there that will validate or verify what people believe or have experienced. I caution against having any expectations as to results, despite all the promise cannabis does show to provide exactly this kind of healing. For some. No matter how much power and potential this plant has, nothing cures everything and everyone. I'm passionate about the plant, but am not promising miracles to anyone.

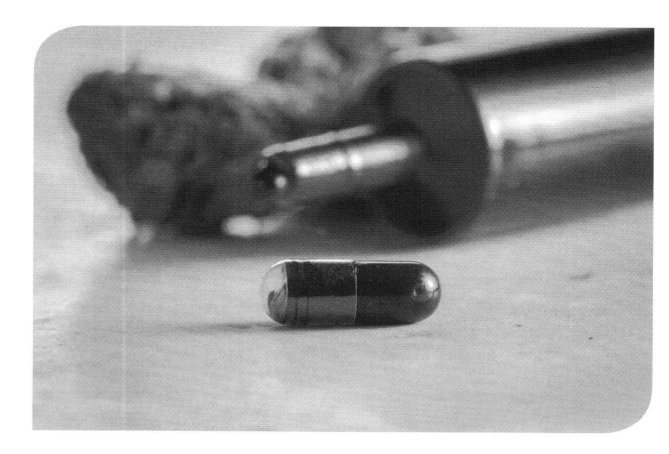

Rick Simpson Oil or RSO is the most widely available, but many other products are being developed which offer the same full-spectrum cannabinoid benefits. This concentrated cannabis oil is quite potent, ranging from 60 to 90% THC (remember that THC kills cancer cells, not brain cells). It is a whole-plant extract with the full spectrum of cannabinoids available in concentrated, bioavailable form. The oil can be orally or rectally administered or applied directly to the skin. Rick Simpson's recommended course of treatment involves building up to very high doses for a 90-day treatment regimen; smaller treatment courses can also be followed.

As I've said, we are all snowflakes—what works for you may not be the same as what works for others. Do your research and follow a process, and you'll be on the best path to the best outcome for you. Interested in a deeper dive? We'll get a bit more into how cannabis oil can be used and how to make it later in the book.

DON'T BELIEVE THE HYPE

Do not buy into the snake-oil pitches of hemp-based CBD oils for curing cancer and taking on serious medical conditions. They can be beneficial, don't get me wrong, but they are not going to take on serious disease like cancer. Only cannabis can deliver the full spectrum of the cannabinoids—every one of which is needed. Be aware that there are a lot of sleazy businesses riding the CBD wave and taking advantage of uninformed and desperate people who are looking for any possible solution to a terrible situation.

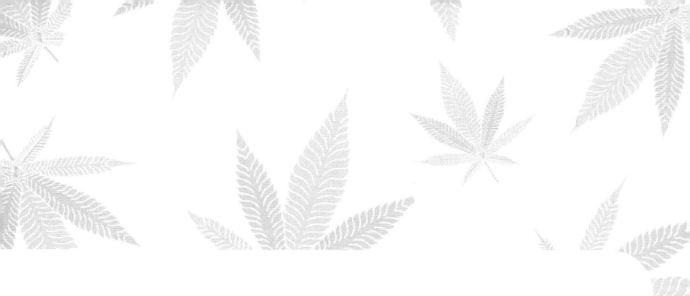

Aren't concentrates like the crack of cannabis?

Concentrates are not to be feared, and can be a healthy and efficient way to consume weed. Extracted cannabis provides you with all those good cannabinoids, just in a more concentrated form. Which means a conscious cannabis consumer actually needs to consume less weed to get the same effects. For patients, concentrates and cannabis oil can be incredibly effective ways to medicate and deliver large amounts of cannabinoids into their systems. Concentrates are not crack. Relax.

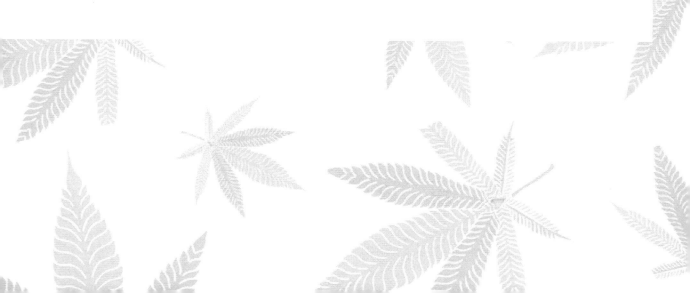

GETTING STARTED: HOW TO CONSUME WITH CONFIDENCE (OR, HOW TO NOT TO FEEL LIKE A CLUELESS OLD FART)

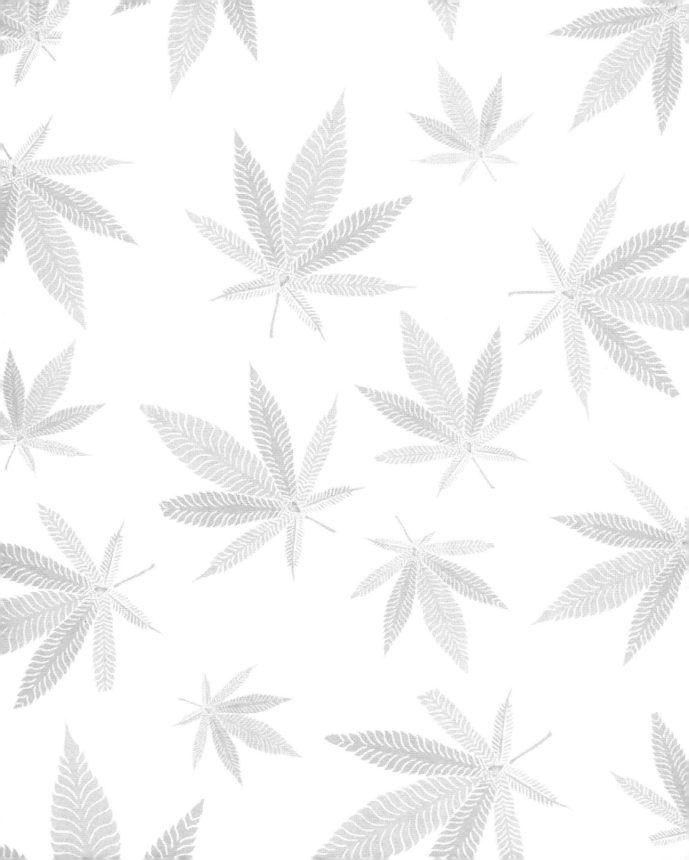

15 | (HAVE FUN) FINDING WHAT WORKS FOR YOU

I've given you a lot of general direction throughout the book, which is the best I can do until we can have a one-on-one conversation to dig further into your unique context. It's a good starting point, but it's also important to remember that every strain has its own cannabinoid profile and every person has their own endocannabinoid system—the Entourage Effect affects everyone in its own unique way. How cannabis is consumed shapes the effects it delivers. And every person has their own preferences and priorities in terms of the experience desired.

It's not about what's best, but what's best for you. Everyone has their own threshold when it comes to getting high. Some love it. Some hate it. (And remember, you don't have to feel high in today's cannabis landscape. There are plenty of options on the spectrum of psychoactivity.)

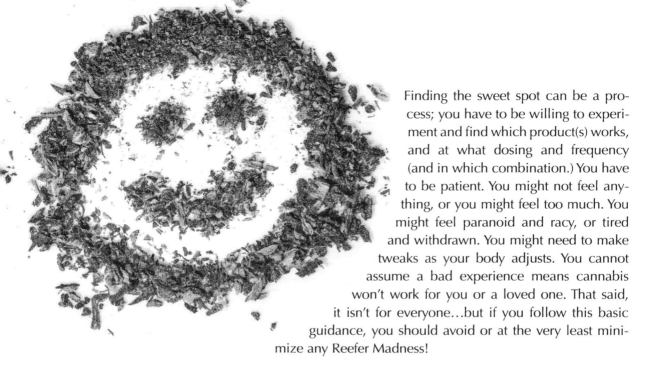

Finding the sweet spot can be a process; you have to be willing to experiment and find which product(s) works, and at what dosing and frequency (and in which combination.) You have to be patient. You might not feel anything, or you might feel too much. You might feel paranoid and racy, or tired and withdrawn. You might need to make tweaks as your body adjusts. You cannot assume a bad experience means cannabis won't work for you or a loved one. That said, it isn't for everyone…but if you follow this basic guidance, you should avoid or at the very least minimize any Reefer Madness!

Low and Slow is the Way to Go

Until you find your threshold and what works for you, the rule of thumb is start low and go slow. You wouldn't tell someone who doesn't drink to start off doing shots. Strains are more potent than ever, concentrates often have potency in 60–80% ranges and edibles can take up to four hours to kick in. Weed can be a creeper, with some strains' effects coming on subtly and stealthily until you're suddenly knocked out. And, the biggest pothead can have an itty bitty edibles tolerance.

There are more and more products coming onto the market targeted to the new user or those who prefer a lighter, more manageable experience. From microdosed mints to 1:1 THC:CBD vape pens, you can stay within the rails by minimizing impairment and mitigating side effects like anxiety, lethargy and spaciness. Don't jump into the deep end—you have the equivalent of floaties to keep you out of trouble.

No matter what or how you're consuming, tune in and listen to your body. Start off microdosing. See how it works with your body's chemistry. You can always consume more. You cannot however, uneat or uninhale what has already passed into your system.

Enjoying Your Edibles
(Or, How Not to Lose a Day or More of Your Life)

In its unactivated form, THC has no psychoactivity—it requires both heat (through a process called decarboxylation) and fat for your digestive system to process it. When ingested, it is transformed within the liver into a drug twice as strong as when it's inhaled. And it's not just stronger; it lasts longer. A lot longer. I know people who have been taken out for an entire weekend by a single edible. Until you know how you process THC through your bloodstream and liver, eating edibles can be a bit like Russian roulette. And if you don't know the dosing or have confidence in its consistency (common with homemade edibles), that gun has more than one bullet in it.

Standard dosing is 10 mg of THC, but newbies, lightweights and cautious canna-consumers should start with 5 mg or even less. In regulated markets with clear labeling requirements, control over dosing is easier, though labeling from market to market is still not always consistent or reliable. Even professional producers have difficulty meeting the advertised dose in their products; and without meticulous testing, it's possible an edible's potency doesn't match the label. Labeling can be unclear and inconsistent. And, if you're eating a homemade edible, dosing is particularly challenging with no testing and potential inconsistency even within the batch itself.

Time for uptake depends on a host of factors, from the type of cannabinoid infusion and solubility to what's in your belly and how long it's been in there before the cannabinoid caravan arrives. Rich and dense products like brownies and chocolate take longer to digest than infused drinks and tinctures. Sucking on a hard candy or lollipop for hours will deliver a slow and steady effect, whereas a single swallow of a gummy or a truffle can flood your system with a wave of cannabinoids. And, sublingual absorption bypasses the liver and goes straight into the bloodstream for the most efficient uptake.

Most people start to feel the effects around 45 minutes or so into the experience—but again, for some people it can take two hours or more. And remember that tinctures and sprays take effect faster than edibles that go into your belly and through your liver, so 15–20 minutes might find you starting

take it

low & slow!

to feel more relaxed. You'll know it's starting to kick in when you feel a pleasant tingling and sense of relaxation.

In higher dosages, edibles can create strong body effects coupled with an almost psychedelic head high. Get too high and it can turn to paranoia and even hallucinations, along with a host of other uncomfortable and unpleasant symptoms like nausea, raciness and fainting. Smaller doses yield milder and, for most people, far more comfortable effects like euphoria, contentedness and relaxation. Effects last roughly six to eight hours, but can go on longer.

Particularly in the beginning, plan for home-based activities like watching a movie or listening to music—you may not feel like socializing, walking around or being someplace loud and energetic.

HOW MUCH SHOULD I DOSE?

According to a recent study in the *Journal of Alcohol and Drug Dependence*, the optimum dose of cannabis, enough to allow the average person to relax, is a paltry 7.5 milligrams. Just a little more—12.5 milligrams, to be precise—greatly increases the chance of experiencing stress and anxiety, which kind of defeats the purpose of using weed to take the edge off in the first place.

What does 7.5 milligrams mean from a canna-newb's perspective? Less than a couple of puffs on a joint. A nibble of an edible. Most people are medicating at much higher levels than needed to achieve the optimal high. For people who've gotten high and anxious, don't assume that bad experience automatically comes with cannabis. It doesn't have to if you proceed with awareness and care.

More products are becoming available for lower dosing, as today's cannabis consumer doesn't seek to get as f'ed up as possible and trends like microdosing start to become mainstream. (More on microdosing later; it's all the rage these days among the entrepreneurial and creative set. For good reason!)

It should be noted that this is one study, and done with THC capsules (versus using plant material), and so it doesn't take into effect the total cannabinoid profile of the plant and the Entourage Effect it delivers. It also doesn't take into account our unique selves. So, to keep repeating myself: it all depends.

Have plenty of non-medicated munchies around to avoid too many nibbles and taking yourself over the edge by mistake. Edibles are more of a body-high effect, and can induce a deep sleep. If you have issues with staying asleep, an edible before bed may help you get a good night's rest—night sweats be damned!

As I've mentioned, many people have had horrific experiences with edibles because they didn't know their limit and obey the rules that have now become standard guidance. If you buy an edible and don't get guidance from your budtender as a newbie to cannabis (more on that shortly; your budtender experience can also be like Russian roulette), you are not buying from a responsible provider.

People with pain, take note: long-term use of painkillers can impact your liver function, which can also impact how it processes THC and other cannabinoids. Edibles may be less effective for people with a liver that is not functioning at peak levels, though apparently levels do stabilize after stopping painkillers. In addition, there are some people who simply don't get high from edibles; hundreds of milligrams leave them completely unaffected.

And, while edibles may be strong compared to inhaled cannabis, they actually deliver a smaller concentration of cannabinoids to the bloodstream. After passing through your digestive system and liver, ingesting edibles gets you only 10 to 20% of THC and other cannabinoids; inhaled cannabis is estimated to deliver closer to 50%, since the cannabinoids go straight to your lungs and into your bloodstream.

Your Nose Knows: Stop and Smell the Flowers

While there is a lot to be said for the ease and simplicity of popping an edible, there is nothing quite like taking in a noseful of dank, delicious weed. With 8,000+ strains and growing, marijuana offers something for everyone, with a vast and varied menu of options. Whether for different taste profiles or for specific cannabinoid therapies, there is a vast world of weed waiting to be explored. Think of it like Goldilocks: this one is too stony, this one is too light, but oh my, THIS one is just right!

If you're buying flower and have choice in strains, let your body do the choosing. Get a big noseful of that weed and find which one you're most drawn to—your body intuitively knows what it wants, and the terpenes in cannabis can help you sniff out a strain you're likely to like. If you're serious about it, take notes. Pay attention to which strains make you feel creative and energetic, which ones give you focus, and which ones make you relaxed or sleepy. Write down how you feel and, if possible, the percentage of THC and other cannabinoids. If you're looking for precision and managing your medicating, include how much you consumed and how often. (This can also be done if you've transformed flower into a concentrate and are dosing through edibles or tinctures.)

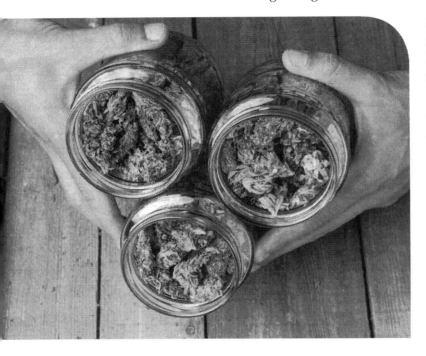

For the newbies or those returning to weed after a long hiatus, take heed: strains are more potent than ever. Until recently when CBD and the other cannabinoids starting getting attention, the only thing most growers cared about was getting the most THC possible into every bud and trichome. That's what the market wanted. Now, between the medical applications of full spectrum cannabinoid therapy and the flood of new consumers not seeking stratospheric highs, there are an increasing number of low-THC (with or without CBD) strains and products available. If you're starting out (again), try a 1:1 THC/CBD product or a low-THC/high-CBD strain and see where that takes you.

Remember, it's less about the specific strains and more about the cannabinoid and terpene profile that works for you. Being able to describe to a budtender or caregiver what kind of effect you're seeking, what types of strains have worked for you in the past (or haven't for that matter) and the kinds of smells and tastes that appeal to you will help get you to the strain(s) most likely to hit your sweet spot.

If you're visiting (or living in) a legal state, it can be tempting to overbuy; after all, it is quite literally like being a kid in a medicated candy store. I hear stories all the time from drivers who are gifted ridiculous amounts of weed from tourists who didn't go on a crazy cannabis binge after all and can't bring their stash home with them. Be sensible. Generally speaking you can always go back for more!

If You Don't Want to Get High (Or If You Do...)

That doesn't mean you can't have THC. It's about psychoactivity and how much or little of it you want. THC has gotten a bad rap; while CBD has rightfully garnered its share of the spotlight, there's a lot of good stuff packed into this little molecule. And, as I've also shown you, there are plenty of ways to get the benefits of THC with no to little psychoactivity, if that's not your thing. Topicals are an easy entry for many with no psychoactivity and immediate localized relief. 1:1 balanced ratios of THC to CBD will deliver a clear, functional high without couchlock, confusion or cloudiness. And if THC just isn't your jam (or isn't legally available to you), that's okay, because CBD-only products are becoming more readily available by the day.

NO HIGH	LOW TO MID HIGH	SUPER HIGH
CBD-only edibles	Low-THC strains	High-THC strains
CBD-only tinctures	High-CBD strains	Concentrates
CBD-only concentrates	1:1 THC/CBD products	Dabbing
Non-THC transdermals	Microdosing	High-THC edibles
Topicals	CBD-rich edibles	High-THC tinctures
Suppositories	CBD/THC tinctures	THC crystalline
	Transdermal patches	
	CBD anything	

Whatever you want from the experience, cannabis can deliver it. But remember that it's a relationship. You've got to date around to find what you like. You have to treat her with respect. You have to be patient and willing to experiment. But, guess what? In this world, you can be poly-cannabis, so to speak! The versatility and the range of ways it can be used makes cannabis the girl you want to take out on the town and can also take home to Mother. You can even pass her around. She can make you feel better. Help you relax and sleep. Take away your pain. Make you laugh. Make you think. Make you forget. Whatever you want, cannabis may just be the gal for you.

If You're High and Don't Like It

On the weed parabola, there can be a lovely ride up and gentle crest back down, but there can also be a steep rise and suddenly you're riding a wave far bigger than you anticipated. You might feel confused, unable to move or talk; you could feel like you're floating away from your body and even hallucinate. You've gone beyond trippy in a fun way and are into deep waters.

Relax. You won't die. (No one ever has, remember?) You might feel like you will. You might want to. But you won't. So take some deep breaths and refer to this section for some easy ways to bring yourself back from the brink if you take in a little too much THC.

If you've been vaporizing or smoking, it will be a short ride. Remember, effects from inhaling come on fast but do not stick around too long. At most, you have an hour before you start to come down. This is one reason newbies to cannabis should start with a vape pen or something manageable and easy. Simply stop puffing. It's really that easy.

If you have CBD or a high-CBD product on hand, that will tame the high and bring you back down quickly. There are products specifically formulated as rescue remedies, but since CBD is something I think is good for everything, having a CBD vape pen or tincture on hand can provide quick relief if your high gets a little out of hand.

If you were impatient with your edibles or overshot the landing pad in terms of your dosing for any reason, try to have no fear. It will all be okay, you just need to hang on and keep telling yourself that you are not dying and that it will pass. If you've followed my guidance and have CBD on hand, take that. Otherwise, you might have some common things around your house that could help...remember your lesson in terpenes? They can be used to tailor a high and tame anxiety as much as their cousins the cannabinoids can.

> **Here are a few handy tricks that could pull you out of a bind:**
>
> **Suck down some lemon juice with a little zest (limonene)**
>
> **Eat some pistachios or pine nuts (pinene)**
>
> **Sniff or crunch on a few black peppercorns/cracked black pepper (beta-caryophyllene)**
>
> **Sniff some pine essential oil or apply topically**

All you have to do is wait it out. Do not drive or try to take on any heavy activities. Take a walk or a cold shower. Lie down. Watch something entertaining. Listen to relaxing music and rest. It will all be okay, and before long you'll have a good story about that time you got so high you thought the cat was judging you. (Of course it's a cat, so it probably was.)

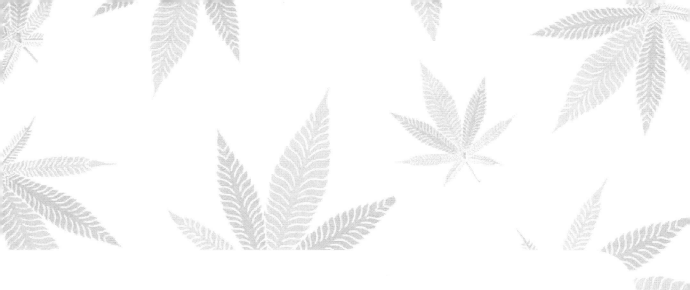

CLOSING QUESTION:

How do I know what and how much I should take?

It all depends—on what you're consuming, how strong it is, how you're consuming it, your physiology, your environment and a host of other factors. The key is to take it low and slow, particularly when it comes to edibles. If you're concerned with getting too high, start with smoking or vaping to keep your experience controllable, and use products with CBD. You will need to experiment to find the strain, product, dosing and timing that work best for you—we are all different and weed is not one-size-fits-all!

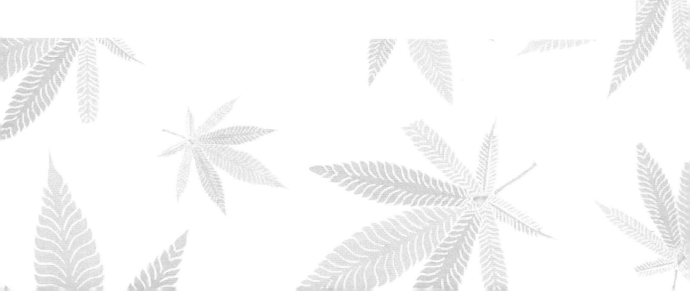

16 | MAKING THE BUY (TRENCHCOAT NOT REQUIRED)

Depending on where you live, you have different options for getting your hands on weed, and different weed options in every state. Every legal state has its own laws and regulations, and its own conditions for medical marijuana laws. Some states have CBD-focused laws and access; others put significant restrictions on the form in which patients can use it. For those of you with legal access to cannabis, depending on the state, you may have medical and recreational dispensaries (often in the same location, but with different products, check-in procedures, limits and regulations for each side), collectives, caregivers and even delivery services available. Every state has its own regulations and products, brands and culture.

In 2018, in the states of Colorado, Oregon, Washington, Alaska, Nevada, Massachusetts, Maine, and California, you should be able to walk into a dispensary, prove you are a legal adult and walk out with a whole lotta weed. (And if you're in the District of Columbia, while weed is technically legal, you cannot buy it anywhere—there is no medical or recreational market in D.C.)

Walking into a dispensary may feel overwhelming (read on for guidance on how to be more comfortable and confident walking into one), but aside from lines of people waiting for their turn, the process is a breeze. Some dispensaries may still feel a like a sketchy Times Square storefront, but more and more of them are becoming as sophisticated and state-of-the-art in terms of customer experience and branding as retailers like Apple and Versace, as efficient and accessible as Walmart or as welcoming as a neighborhood apothecary.

If it's the stigma and judgment you fear, that is likely more in your head than in reality. People's eyes have opened to cannabis and its value and potential. Attitudes have relaxed. The image of pot has been elevated from stoner stereotype to sophisticated consumption with intent. Not everywhere and not by everyone, but the vast majority of Americans now approve of its legalization and safe access for adults. Don't let fear, shame or embarrassment stand in the way of feeling better.

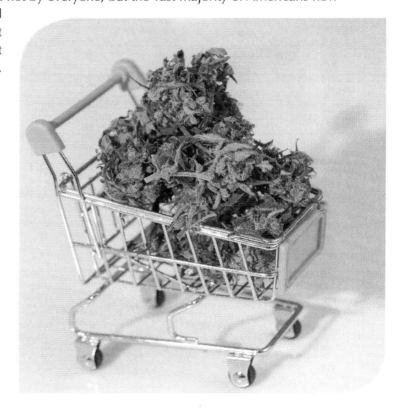

Getting Carded: This Time It's Not For Show

In states where medical marijuana is available, getting a card gets you access (and legal protection.) For some, a card is the only option to get cannabis. For others, it's a choice, offering far better selection and variety of products, higher dosing and bigger limits, as well as lower costs (and oftentimes, shorter lines!) Medical products are taxed at lower rates and often priced lower/have better overall value. And, generally speaking, budtenders serving medical patients are more knowledgeable about a broad range of conditions and the products that can help.

The steps are simple, but the process may not be easy. It all depends on the state. Some require no real documentation; others are more rigorous in their process, with only a small group of authorized doctors who must vet patients. For example, in Florida, it's required that you've tried "mainstream" treatments before seeking medical marijuana. And yes, it does put you into the state's system. While I don't suspect it will ever be an issue, for those with reservations about "the man," this may be a legitimate barrier. Or for those who have to register with a state board of health or have government positions; marijuana may be legal in your state, but that doesn't mean you can't still get in trouble for it professionally, even with a card.

Every state has its own system—in California for example, it can be done entirely online—but the basic process goes something like this:

1 Consult with a qualified healthcare provider

Now, because every state is different, this may be as easy as meeting with your primary care provider, or it can require finding and making an appointment with an authorized physician and providing rigorous documentation. Even in states where every physician can write a recommendation, not every physician will. And even doctors who are opening their eyes to cannabis' medical and therapeutic potential don't know much about it, unless they've gone through training or taken it upon themselves to learn.

In many cases, it's easier to get a recommendation outside of the traditional healthcare system. Don't fret! You can use the google to find medical cannabis doctors, clinics and wellness centers focused exclusively on seeing patients for medical marijuana evaluations. Doctors and clinics trained to work with medical marijuana patients and their conditions are on the front lines and are seeing what's working every day. (And they know how to work the system, so it puts far less burden on you to navigate the process once you've had your evaluation. As with everything, do your homework and choose a reputable provider—there are definitely some skeevy operations that may be legit, but are also ones I wouldn't want to send Mom to, y'know?)

Every state has its own conditions for which medical marijuana is approved, and new conditions may be added so be sure to do your homework to know what is and is not in scope before scheduling a consultation. While cannabis should be legally available for pain management everywhere, it isn't. California has a long list of conditions, but most states are far more restrictive. If you don't know what options are available in your state, go to the National Cannabis Industry Association's website (thecannabisindustry.org) and use the interactive map to see the market and regulations state by state.

2 Get a written authorization/recommendation
The physician must verify that you have a qualifying health condition that will benefit from medical marijuana, in whatever bureaucratic format is required by the state. Note this is not an actual prescription for cannabis; you will not get a piece of paper from a tear-off pad that you can take to your local pharmacy. You will not need to get a recommendation every time you want to use medical marijuana; but you will need to renew on a regular basis.

3 Apply for your card
Along with whatever medical authorization is needed, there will be other forms and documentation (photos, fingerprints—it all depends on the state) to include verifying your residency, identity and such. There's also the ability to assign a caregiver for medical patients, which of course requires more paperwork. And fees, there are always fees. Send everything in and assuming there are no hiccups in the process, you can expect to receive a card in the mail anywhere from 30 to 90 days later, on average. Once you have card in hand (most states won't accept temporary paperwork), you're ready to start shopping!

Be a Savvy Shopper and Shape Your Experience

You shouldn't be afraid of walking into a dispensary. There is plenty of security and safety, no matter where it's located. You've read the book (or at least skimmed through it), so by now you should feel confident in knowing what effects you're looking for and how to find products and strains that might work for you.

This is important. Not just so you're not flying blind, but even with help from the most intuitive waiter or sommelier, you still need to know what you enjoy, what you don't want or what doesn't work for you and what kind of experience you want. Imagine how frustrating it is to be asked what to recommend with no input or direction whatsoever. It's kind of like when my mom says she needs computer help but cannot give me one problem or thing she wants to do. It's frustrating for both of us. (But me, really it's frustrating for me.) And so it's safe to assume if you have no clue what you want, a budtender is going to fall back on what they like, or what they're trying to move that day. Take an active role in the conversation or you truly are playing Russian roulette with what you might get.

It's your responsibility to define, shape and control the experience as best you can. From dosing to what might work best for you (or a loved one; I assume they are interchangeable terms in this conversation), no one knows you better than you. There are a lot of great budtenders who will help you find exactly what you're looking for; but there are equally as many well-intentioned but untrained workers who don't really know what they're talking about, especially when talking to people outside their demographic bubble. Marijuana may be medicine, but there is no required training for budtenders.

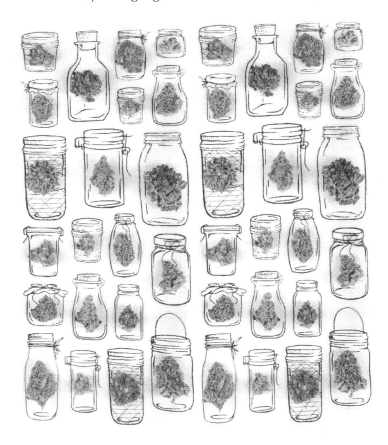

My personal experience with budtender knowledge and service has been all over the board. Most of them truly do seem to care, but there is a vast range of expertise out there. When I was searching for an edible to help me transition off painkillers and was struggling to find one that worked for me, it was only after weeks (and hundreds of dollars) trying different products that a budtender (who wasn't even serving me; he happened to overhear my inquiry and piped in) asked if I had been taking opioids for an extended period of time. When I said I was just coming off them, he advised that my liver likely wasn't processing the edibles and it was all pretty much a waste until my function returned to normal levels. That certainly would have been helpful to know far sooner, and had he not been in the right place at the right time, I might have kept beating my head against the wall. Instead, I stuck with inhalation and in time, my body stabilized and came back to normal.

I've educated more than a few budtenders during my dispensary experiences and actually enjoy the exchange of knowledge and information. This is an ever-evolving landscape, and even those with deep expertise or training always have more to learn. There's a lot of subjectivity in experience and effects. Every person is different. Strains are different (remember, it's all about the cannabinoid profile).

There should be more training for the men and women on the front lines of cannabis, not just about the weed itself, but about the people using it and how best to help them. But until the industry catches up with best practices in other retail and healthcare experiences, or until you find your go-to budtender who knows just what you need, it's on you to identify what you want and which types of cannabis products are likely to work. Be prepared, but be open about your newbie status; there's no need to play it cool. Those of us who sling the lingo every day can forget to slow it down and break down the basics—raise a hand, ask questions and don't be afraid to take your time finding what you want. It's your experience. Get the most from it.

> **Remember the slogan for that old store Syms?**
>
> **"An educated consumer is our best customer."**
>
> **Learn it. Know it. Live it.**

Talking Shop
(Or, How Get What You Want and Not Look Like A Rube)

Okay, you have a general sense of what you're looking for and are ready to start shopping. Whether through a budtender or your friendly neighborhood dealer, you'll be asked questions and should have the opportunity to ask yours. What labeling is available and what testing has been done? Is the product grown organically and pesticide-free? For the most part, people who enjoy weed, enjoy talking about weed, so don't be afraid to start a conversation!

Weight: Flower is sold in grams/ounces. In smaller amounts, it tends to be in grams; once you're at a quarter ounce (7 grams) or more, the weight is generally referred to in ounce increments. If you're buying concentrate, you'll want to know that most products are sold as either .5 gram or 1 gram units. Weed is sold as buds (or nugs), but oftentimes you can buy shake, which is all the bits and pieces that fall off in the jar. It's cheaper and can be good for joints and cooking, but it's definitely not the same as good bud.

Quality: Ask if the cannabis was grown without pesticides and if it's been tested. (Obviously not a question to ask the neighborhood weed dealer, but you get the idea.) Technically, cannabis cannot be called organic, since it's not under the umbrella of the FDA. But you want to consume cannabis that's been grown without chemicals, particularly when it's going into your body in a concentrated, extracted form. Don't assume this is the case at all; many large, indoor grows use commercial pesticides to keep crops free of critters, fungus and other icky stuff. Scott's Miracle Gro is already on the market with hydroponics products. If you're getting concentrates, ask what kind of extraction process was used. If you care about

WHAT SHOULD I LOOK FOR IN MY FLOWER?

Good cannabis flowers should have a white crystalline substance on them—this indicates a high trichome content, which generally means you're getting quality stuff. However, watch out for powdery mildew. It's also white and is an indicator of poor quality. Trichome will glisten and look like sugar crystals. Mildew looks like baby powder.

chemicals, choose CO_2 over butane, or go for solventless extractions like rosin or distillate. If you care about the way the food you put into your mouth was grown, you should care about the way the weed you put in your body was grown and processed.

Effects: Be clear on what you want from the experience and what you don't. How do you want to feel? Uplifted? Energetic? Creative? Talkative? The more descriptive you are, the better the recommendation will be. Do you want to feel elevated or are you going for pure body effects? If you don't want to feel high, remember that any product with CBD in it will counter psychoactivity; you can still get the benefits of THC without feeling altered.

Experience: What is the setting for your consumption? Will you be home or out and about? Do you want portability and discretion? Precision control, simplicity and ease? Are you consuming everything at once, or will a single edible carry you for a week? The more context to the kind of experience you're seeking, the better the product recommendations will be.

Let Your Nose Lead the Way

Remember terpenes? These sexy little compounds do the heavy lifting when it comes to the effects you'll feel. Remember, think of sativas and indicas on a spectrum, and use terpenes as a key indicator as to how you're going to feel when all is said and done.

Generally speaking, packaged, processed cannabis products are not strain specific—though concentrates and vape pen cartridges with extracts from a single strain are becoming more available. As consumers and patients demand more specificity and control over their experience, we'll see more choice become available.

IF YOU WANT...	LOOK FOR...	THAT HAVE...	STRAINS LIKE...
Sharper focus (and better breathing)	Sativas and sativa-leaning hybrids	Sharp, sweet aromas of pine, conifers and sage (Pinene)	Jack Herer Blue Dream OG Kush Dutch Treat
Uplifted spirits and energy	Sativas and sativa-leaning hybrids	Smells of citrus, juniper and peppermint (Limonene)	Sour Diesel Super Lemon Haze Trainwreck Green Crack
Less of an appetite and less pain	Sativa-leaning hybrids	Woody, earthy aromas of hops and coriander (Humulene)	Sour Diesel Headband OG Kush Girl Scout Cookies
Relaxation and sedation	Indicas and indica-leaning hybrids	Musky and herbal with citrus notes; think bay leaves and lemongrass (Myrcene)	Blue Dream Grandaddy Purple Northern Lights Alien OG
Less anxiety and a better night's sleep	Indicas and indica-leaning hybrids	Smells of lavender, citrus and spice (Linalool)	Lavender Skywalker OG Headband Pink Kush
Less pain and inflammation	Indicas and indica-leaning hybrids	Peppery and spicy aromas like in oregano and basil (Caryophyllene)	Girl Scout Cookies Bubba Kush OG Kush Chemdawg

Come Along on a Fantastic Voyage

There are as many dispensaries in some legal states as there are Starbucks. And there's pretty much a Starbucks on every block these days.... Every dispensary is different, offering its own mix of products, strains of cannabis and overall customer experience. There are chains aspiring to become the Walmart of weed, and high-end boutiques with a highly curated selection and top-notch customer service. Depending on what's important to you, there's likely a dispensary out there for you.

If word of mouth is an option, ask around to see which dispensaries other people like, and why. Go online or download an app like Weedmaps to see what's available in your area and what people have to say about their experience and the products. Is the staff knowledgeable and approachable? If you're a patient, see what kind of programs they offer; many dispensaries offer a lot of support to their patients. Does it have a good selection? Is it clean and safe? With so many options becoming available, don't just randomly pick the first dispensary you see. Look around for deals and offers. There are even websites focused specifically on aggregating deals in different areas.

Be prepared to be overwhelmed by choice: every dispensary carries different products and strains, but generally speaking you will have to make some choices. Remember when everyone first walked into Willie Wonka's Chocolate Factory? It's kind of like that, except you can't actually eat or drink anything on site. And definitely don't lick anything. But you will be blown away by the variety and creativity: just about every kind of chocolate and candy you can imagine, taffy, bacon brittle, vegan pot capsules, root beer, coffee, massage oil, pens with transdermal creams (that smell fantastic, in some cases)!

And remember, in some states, you don't even have to leave the comfort of your home—a small version of the dispensary can be brought right to your door. However, until you've got your weed legs, so to speak, you might want some hand-holding and guidance from a pro.

Other Ways to Get Your Hands on Some Weed

Perhaps you live in a state without legal access, or don't have a qualifying medical condition in a state that has medical marijuana access; or for whatever reasons, getting marijuana through the system isn't an option for you. What are your options?

For the record, by no means do I encourage or endorse illegal activity. I cannot advocate for you to break the law. Where legal access is available, use it. If you've got a green thumb, grow it.

But if you were to ask me for advice on how to score some weed, I would first suggest you ask whomever turned you on to this book—it's a pretty sure bet. You might ask your kids (double bonus if they gave you this book). It seems more parents than kids are getting lifted these days, but there are a growing number of young adults choosing cannabis over alcohol as a safer and more mindful alternative. I'm giving you a conversation guide to help you talk to your family and friends about weed—it's the perfect opportunity to ask if anyone can hook you up.

Alternatively, a discreet (or direct, depending on your style) inquiry with your hairstylist, massage therapist, young, hip neighbor or other friend in the service industry could get you a trustworthy and safe cannabis connection. And more than likely, it's far from a dark, back-alley drug deal. There are delivery services and high-end procurers of the finest cannabis available. There are people who grow their own medicine and small collectives of patients who are taking care of their needs in the best way for them.

Places NOT to buy marijuana: Craigslist (and the internet in general), a head shop or other store where they sell stuff for use with weed or the guy hanging out at the park.

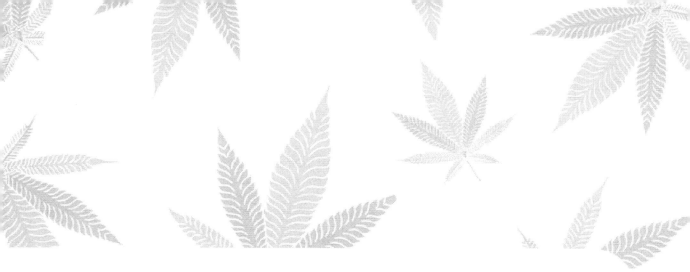

CLOSING QUESTION:

What's it like to buy weed—does it feel like walking into an adult video store?

You don't need a trenchcoat and you don't need to feel like you're walking into a seedy, sketchy situation. Dispensaries are becoming high-end, consumer-driven retail shops. Security and safety are prime directives for any business operating in this industry. But, you do need to be prepared when you make the buy—have some sense of what effects or products you are seeking, as well as what you don't want. Do help the guy or gal helping you out and take an active role in your purchase; it will help you have the best experience. And do have fun with shopping, it's a whole new world of weed out there....go check it out!

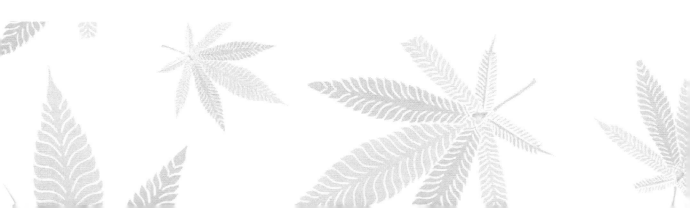

17 | THE BEGINNER'S GUIDE TO CONSUMPTION

Okay, so you've made the buy (or skipped that step because you had friends or family hook you up.) Now what? Let's go over some basic how-to's, tips and etiquette to help you get comfortable with the actual consumption of weed.

If You Want to Smoke a Joint...

I hope you bought a pre-roll, because rolling your own joint is a bitch to learn. I've been smoking weed for 20+ years and I still can't roll one. Even with lessons. My joints look like sad little flabby twigs.

I'll give you the basics for rolling a joint, but in my opinion, you're not going to learn to roll a fattie by looking at a diagram. So I'll also give you my tip: buy cones (pre-formed joints you pack instead of roll) and make joints that way. It's much easier.

You'll need:

Flower	Papers or cones
A grinder	A tray/surface to catch the random bits and pieces of weed

Grind the flower and sprinkle into your paper or cone. If you're rolling a joint, use the diagram as a guide and good luck to you!

If using a cone, you can use the side of the grinder to help scoop the weed into the opening. Your cones probably came with a little plastic or cardboard straw—use that to gently pack the weed in. Continue until it's full and tamped down, but not so tight that air can't get through. (This holds true for joints: tighter is not better for a good smoking experience.)

Twist the tip to keep all the ground up goodness from spilling out, grab a lighter and fire up. Take a small puff, inhale and release. And you might be surprised to know you don't need to hold your hit. Many of us have been told to hold our hits for as long as possible, but in actuality, all that will do is make you more likely to cough. THC and cannabinoids are absorbed into your lungs in less than a second; any longer is just holding your breath. You can expand your lungs to provide as much real estate as possible to absorb the cannabinoids, but exhale as soon as you've taken your full breath.

Start small and take it slow to begin. Have something to sip on in case you do end up with a coughing fit. You may need to re-light the joint off and on, depending on how quickly it's burning and actively it's being hit. If you're smoking with a group, the general rule is "puff, puff, pass." Don't bogart the joint while others are waiting.

And remember, no one likes a slobberer. Keep the tip dry!

How to Roll a Joint
a step-by-step guide

STEP 1:
GRIND CANNABIS

If you don't have a grinder, use scissors or break up flower with fingertips.

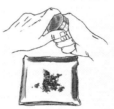

STEP 2:
MAKE A FILTER (AKA A CRUTCH)

Use the cardboard filters that come with rolling papers (or a business card). Make a few accordion folds and then roll into a filter tip.

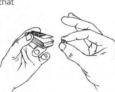

STEP 3:
FILL PAPER WITH CANNABIS

Hold paper lengthwise with sticky part facing you. Place crutch on the left side (if righty, reverse if lefty) and hold while sprinkling flower into the crease (1/2 - 1 gram on average). Form and shape the joint.

STEP 4:
ROLL & PACK JOINT

Using your thumbs and forefingers, pinch the paper in between your fingertips and roll back and forth.

Keep rolling until you've packed it into its final shape. It should be tight enough to hold its shape and loose enough to enable air flow.

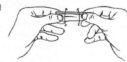

STEP 5: FINISH & SEAL

This is where it can fall apart, literally. Tuck the unglued side of the paper into the roll, lick the gummy edge and roll upward into the sticky gum.

Tack down one end of the paper (crutch side) and work your way down the rest of the seam by tucking and sealing the joint from end to end.

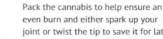

STEP 6: ENJOY!

Pack the cannabis to help ensure an even burn and either spark up your joint or twist the tip to save it for later.

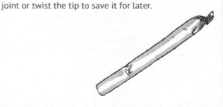

If You Want to Smoke a Bowl (in a Pipe or Bong)...

The basic function is the same for both—you pack a bowl with ground-up weed. That bowl is either in a pipe or one-hitter, or is a separate piece that gets inserted into a bong filled with water (and perhaps a little ice for further cooling of the smoke, if that floats your boat.) Technically, a bong is illegal since it's drug paraphernalia, so it's officially referred to as a water pipe in head shops and such.

You'll need:

Flower   A pipe or bong

Break off/crumble a bit of the flower and sprinkle it into your bowl. It doesn't need to be ground like it does for a joint, but it does need to be broken up. You may want to put a screen in between the bowl and the weed—there's a little hole at the bottom of the bowl, and sometimes ash and weed bits get sucked through as you finish the bowl. Don't jam too much in there—and if you're just going to take a couple of hits, just put in a little nug or two. Fresh weed is always better than partially smoked leftovers later.

Let's start with a pipe. See if it has a hole on the side—this is a carb. You put your finger over it when you light the bowl and start to inhale, and remove it for a big hit (or you can keep your finger over the carb on the first hit, exhale and then finish up whatever smoke is in the chamber with a second inhale and removal of your finger from the carb.) If there's a carb and it's uncovered, you won't get any suction or airflow.

If you're using a bong, the first rule of thumb is never blow; always suck. Blowing will result in a big bowl of wet weed. And that makes everyone sad. Make sure not to overfill the chamber with water, or you will get backsplash when drawing the smoke through the chamber. Not so bad the first time or two, but that water can get pretty nasty. A mouthful of bongwater on the tail end of a sesh will make you very unhappy indeed. Too little water, and all you'll get is air without any water filtration. You'll know the level is too low if there's no bubbling when you inhale.

HOW LONG SHOULD YOU HOLD YOUR HIT?

Actually, you don't. All it will do for you is make you cough. Everything is absorbed within seconds—so what you want is maximum exposure to the receptors in your lungs. So, take a big inhale to expand your lungs, and then exhale right away.

Catch your breath and then put your mouth over the top, light the weed and inhale comfortably. (You can have someone else light the bowl for you if you want to focus on your inhalation.) Not all bongs have a carb, because the bowl and its placement in the bong provide the same suction effect without needing to use your finger. With a bong, the water will cool the smoke, making for a far less harsh hit. But it can also deceive you into taking a bigger hit than you can handle, so tread carefully. You can take a few smaller hits without removing the bowl or releasing the carb, or once you've got a nice milky-white chamber of smoke in the bong, pull up the bowl and inhale deeply (exhaling without holding).

If you're going to cough, do not cough into the bong! If you feel like you're going to cough, remove your mouth from the bong. Either cough or wait it out. The general rule of etiquette is to always clear the chamber before passing to the next person; the stale leftover smoke is often called a buffalo fart and is a faux pas in some stoner circles. But if you don't let it get stale and someone wants to share it, by all means don't let it go to waste! Otherwise, remove the carb and blow any remaining smoke out of the chamber to clear it before passing it along. Do you best not to knock over the bong; it happens, but it's most definitely a party foul.

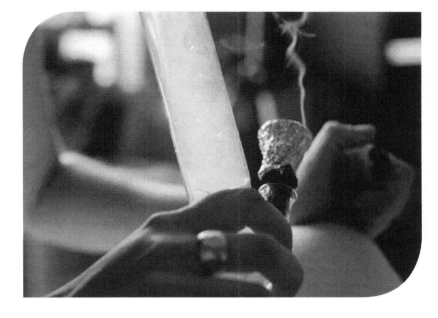

Bongs (aka "water pipes") come in every imaginable shape and size. There's even bubblers, which are like a small bong or large pipe with water filtration. Generally made from glass, acrylic, bamboo, or ceramic, they range from fairly inexpensive to incredibly pricey. A word of advice: when buying a glass bong, don't start with the prettiest or most expensive one. I can't count how many bongs I've broken by knocking them over or dropping them. Consider your klutziness when making any investment in your gear—I am notorious for not being able to have nice things.

Keep your water fresh and you won't have to clean your bong as often. But you will need to clean both a hand pipe or water pipe on occasion; there are plenty of cleaning products on the market, or you can do it yourself with a few simple items like isopropyl alcohol, dish soap, coarse salt and a plastic bag.

1 Soak the gunky piece in hot water and dish soap for bit to loosen everything up. Give it a really good rinse.

2 Get a good handful of coarse salt and either throw it into a bag with the pipe or into the chamber of the bong.

3 Fill the bag or chamber with a good amount of alcohol (submerge the pipe or gunk in the chamber) and seal up the opening(s.) Use your hands and fingers to block up any holes.

4 Shake it vigorously. Repeat. And repeat again. Pretend you're on a commercial for the Shake Weight. Do this for at least five minutes.

5 Empty and rinse. The longer you've gone without cleaning, the longer this will take. You might need to do it more than once. Or you might want to just go buy something new!

You can also use pipe cleaners soaked in alcohol to clean stems and other parts with smaller openings.

If You Want to Vape...

These days, vaporizing is on just about everyone's list. It's easy on the lungs and easy to consume, manageable and controllable—and it doesn't stink up the place. There are a gazillion options and growing. You can use a desktop vaporizer or take it on the go. You can use flower or concentrate. You can do it yourself or buy something packaged and ready to go.

Devices are getting ever more sophisticated and subtle, with features like precision temperatures and dosing and designs that look like lipsticks and pens. I have vaped in front of people without anyone knowing, and picked up a vape pen thinking it was actually a pen—and it's only going to get more functional and more integrated into the real world.

I'm not sure if it's the chicken or the egg when it comes to choosing whether to get a vaporizer for flower or concentrate. Think about how and what you will be consuming for the most part. What do you have access to? Will you be mostly at home or taking it out and about? Do you want something plug-and-play?

A portable vape pen is the easiest jumping-off point. You don't have to do anything other than perhaps screw a cartridge into the battery and inhale. Perhaps you have to press a button, but most likely not. Most pens separate the oil cartridge from the battery, so you can recharge and replace the cartridge when it's empty. You can also swap cartridges to change up what you're vaping. You might want a sativa to start the day and then an indica in the evening to wind down and get a good night's sleep. Some pens are disposable—by no means single use, but after some period of time, depending on how much you're hitting it, it dies out and you're done. For light to moderate users, a cartridge can last months at a time.

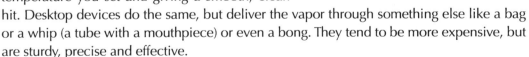

There are a variety of handheld and desktop devices available if you want to vaporize flower. Hand-held devices have a small chamber that serves as an oven, heating the weed to whatever temperature you set and giving a smooth, clean hit. Desktop devices do the same, but deliver the vapor through something else like a bag or a whip (a tube with a mouthpiece) or even a bong. They tend to be more expensive, but are sturdy, precise and effective.

Many vaporizers can handle all forms of weed, from flower to oils and concentrates like rosin and shatter. So if you don't want to choose just one form, look for a vaporizer with versatility.

Remember, there's no combustion with vaping, so there's no lighter required or burning of your weed. You're going to pack whatever you're consuming into your device's chamber, and then follow the instructions that came with it. Draw in—remember, don't hold—and exhale. Suck and blow. It's the easiest, fastest and most manageable way to consume.

IF I WANT TO VAPE, WHAT DO I NEED TO KNOW AND CONSIDER ABOUT VAPORIZERS?

To be honest, I'm a joint gal. I have and have used my fair share of vaporizers, but by no means am I an expert. So, I asked an expert to answer this question. Let me introduce you to my very good friend, Holly, who took a different but similar potrepreneurial path.

Holly founded Healthy Headie Lifestyle, an in-home education and experience model not all that different than the Mary Kay or Tupperware parties we all grew up with. You may have seen her on CBS or, if you're lucky enough to have an interaction with her as she helps patients and consumers at Harborside (the largest dispensary in California) she may actually help you choose the vaporizer that's best for you.

Here's what she had to say about vaping and choosing a vaporizer:

> First of all, there are a lot of differences in vaping, so you have to start with some basic questions. Are you vaporizing flower or concentrate? Do you want a desktop device or something portable? Vaping is not the same as e-cigs, just to be clear.
>
> Vaporizing is different than smoking in that you only inhale the pure vapor of the oils; you're not getting plant material, the stuff that comes with lighting it on fire or even the butane of the flame.
>
> When you vaporize cannabis, it's doesn't have the hammer effect you can get with smoking. You do inhale vapor, but there is no smoke. It's a little more subtle; too subtle for some. But, it does work, even if it doesn't get some people as high as they would like.

By the way, subtle doesn't mean you're not "getting anything." Vaping does give you a lot of advantages, even (or especially) if you don't think it's working. Regardless of the effects, you are still getting cannabinoids into your body.

Your first consideration is price, since devices can range from $60 to $600. (A high-end desktop vaporizer like the Volcano, which has been around for long time and is used by Bill Maher, will run you around $600.)

Think about whether you're vaping at home or on the go. Desktop vaporizers require an outlet and oftentimes offer more power. Portable devices give flexibility, but may not have the power or precision a medical patient or advanced cannabist may want.

Do you want your vaporizer to handle flower, concentrate or both? Some devices only handle one form of consumption; others offer the flexibility to vaporize any form of cannabis.

In general, if you're just getting started or need discretion, get a less expensive hand-held device. If possible, try a friend's vaporizer first. If you dig it and want to get all techie and sophisticated, there are plenty of options to consider and certainly more to come.

If You Want to Eat Your Weed...

Hopefully I've effectively reinforced the wide variability in experience that can be had with edibles. Blind or inconsistent dosing, your individual metabolism, what's in your belly, impatience and a host of other factors can turn a good experience ugly. And no one wants that.

One of the first things to consider is how you're going to be consuming your edible. In one bite? In one sitting? Over the course of a few doses? Will you be sharing it? Taking it on the go with you? I've lost more than a few chocolate bars to a hot car or found bits and pieces stuck to the inside of my purse. Once you get your context clear, you can choose wisely when making your selection.

Even experienced potheads can get taken out by an edible. Jumping in the deep end is never a good idea; dipping a toe in the water to start always is, and even once you know how to swim, you should still enter on the shallow end. Don't get cocky, even once you have a sense of your tolerance and thresholds. A little discipline goes a long way.

HOW MUCH SHOULD I TAKE?

It depends. Are you new to this and a lightweight? Are you comfortable with feeling high? What are you going to be doing? How does your body metabolize marijuana? You will have to find your own dosing range; but for loose guidance, beginners and people with low thresholds should stick to 5–10 mg. More experienced users start with 20–30 mg. Serious stoners and patients in need of higher dosing might go with 50 mg or higher.

It's on you to find the levels that are comfortable and effective for you. Don't just go by what your friend took.

Remember: safety first, people. Don't mix other substances to start. Definitely don't drive. If you have kids or pets running around, make sure you don't leave any treats lying around. All the labeling in the world doesn't matter to a dog or toddler. I've known more than one dog to get through a sealed package. Responsible consumption is more than just taking care of yourself.

FOLLOW THIS GUIDE AND YOU'LL PROTECT YOURSELF FROM, WELL, YOURSELF! NEWBIES STAY STRICT WITH RULE #1; EVERY PERSON SHOULD FOLLOW RULES 2 AND 3 EVERY TIME.

1 **Get low.** No more than 10 mg to start. If you tend to have a low tolerance/high sensitivity, I'd suggest 2.5–5 mg. Remember that dosing is per serving and not per package. I've seen a single cookie or brownie range in potency from 10 mg to 1,000 mg. Put those glasses on and read the label! And if it's homemade or otherwise unclear how much THC is going in your mouth, err on the side of caution. Nibble, don't nosh.

2 **Sit tight.** Be patient. The easiest way to overconsume is to think nothing is happening and go back for more. It can take hours for your liver to do its thing. Wait at least 45 minutes (and up to two hours) before a second dose. If you do go back for more, don't just take another 10 mg—that's doubling your dosing.

3 **Plan ahead.** Nourish yourself first. Avoid the edible sandtrap and have plenty of non-medicated munchies on hand. Edibles are tastier than ever. It's easy to find yourself reaching for just another bite. In this case, one bite too many can lead to far worse repercussions than needing to just loosen your belt buckle. And, think about what kind of edible will be most satisfying and functional—a 50 mg truffle isn't really shareable or easily dosed out in smaller pieces.

If You Want to Dab...

Dabbing is done with concentrates like shatter, wax, budder, live resin, rosin, sugar, sugar wax and even pure terpenes. Dosed responsibly, it's a great way to get the most flavor, aroma and effect from all the cannabinoids and terpenes. As I said earlier, dabbing is not for amateurs. Trying it while under the direction of a dabtender is a safe way to see what it's all about.

At home, dabbing generally requires a rig; essentially a bong, but instead of a bowl, there's a nail which gets superheated by hand via a butane torch or electronically through a ceramic or titanium e-nail. An e-nail is more expensive, but gives you precision—for medical patients or those who get into weed like others get into wine tasting, it may be worth the investment.

You'll need:

  – A dab rig or bong with adapter

  – Heat (butane torch or e-nail)

  – Dabber (metal or ceramic tool to take a dab of concentrate and vaporize on the nail

  – Carb cap (lid for the nail to block airflow, much like on a pipe or bong)

  – Silicone mat (to rest dab tool on; it gets hot and very sticky)

If you're using an e-nail, get it to heated up to whatever temperature you want...generally between 500 and 650 degrees, though lower or higher temperatures can be used. Put water into the glass bubbler to cool the vapor as you inhale.

First get a little bit of concentrate onto the tip of the dabber. A little dab will do ya—don't take a big glob. If it's too big or sticky, use the wax paper or dab mat to get it down to just a wee bit on the tip.

If you're using a torch, heat the bottom of the nail diagonally, with some flame going up the side but most heating the bottom. Heat evenly until the nail is glowing red. Let it cool a bit.

Pick up the dabber with the concentrate loaded on it. Before bringing it to the nail, put your mouth over the opening of the glass and get ready to inhale. Touch the tip of the dabber to the inside of the nail and let the concentrate melt into the bowl and slide down the side. Put the dabber onto the silicone mat. Pull the smoke into your lungs and move away. Cover the nail with the carb cap. You can continue taking pulls until you're done. Remove the carb cap and clear the chamber. Put it on the silicone mat where you also put the dab tool.

Be warned: burns can easily happen with dabbing. Picking up or touching the nail is an easy mistake to make once or twice. Leaving the carb cap on too long will make it searing hot and really painful to remove with your fingers, likely causing you to fling it away from you.

If you're interested in dabbing but don't want to make the investment in a rig, there are portable, hand-held dabbers on the market. They're more involved than a vape pen, but far less so than a rig.

MAKE YOUR OWN ROSIN OIL

Generally speaking, making your own extracts is not the way to go. If you want to consume concentrates, buy them. But there is one extract you can make at home safely and with common household items: rosin oil. Rosin is a pure concentrate of marijuana's medicinal properties, tastier and more potent than flower. It's used for dabbing, and can also be used in some vaporizers.

You can make rosin in three easy steps with just three items: a hair straightener, parchment paper and weed. For the weed, you can use bud or kief to make the oil. One nug will yield a 7–10% rosin oil, enough for one to two decent dabs.

1. Set the straightening iron to medium-low heat.

2. Fold a piece of the parchment paper in half and put some weed in the middle.

3. Insert and squeeze the parchment paper with lots of pressure for about five seconds—open and remove the flattened, heated starting material.

The ring of oily resin is what you're looking for. You can repeat this process two or three times to get more from each small nugget you heat. Use a dabber tool to scrape the oil from the paper, and you're ready to go!

Consume Safely, Responsibly and Enjoyably (Or, Don't Be a Dumbass)

We are all grown-ups, so I shouldn't need to remind you to behave like one when approaching your relationship and experience with cannabis. That is not to say you can't enjoy yourself and have fun exploring the full range of benefits weed might deliver to you or a loved one. But like anything, it should be done in moderation and with intent.

As we've covered, you can't overdose or become addicted to marijuana. The plant in and of itself is safe and harmless. However, you can over dose and put yourself and others in danger by driving, starting to cook something and flaking out, falling asleep with a lit joint in hand, losing your balance or becoming lightheaded and taking a spill. You can lose hours to bliss and relaxation, good for the soul but perhaps not so much for the schedule of a busy mom.

Don't drink alcohol and consume cannabis, especially in the beginning. (Once you are confident in your cannabis consumption, alcohol can be responsibly used in conjunction with weed…there are no interactions. But tread carefully and be aware of how the two work synergistically with your body.) Don't drive when you're high. If you're taking medications, be open with your doctor and have the conversation. Be prepared for resistance and ignorance, but use the opportunity to share what you've learned and perhaps what you've experienced.

And on the topic of medications, much like you wouldn't leave pills just scattered around, the same goes for your weed. Particularly edibles. Dogs will get high. Kids will get high. They will all be okay, but it's scary and uncomfortable for everyone involved. And expensive, should that lapse in judgment lead to a trip to the ER or vet. There are lots of great options that keep your stash safe, and oftentimes smell-proof. Some are elegant pieces that blend right in with your living room accessories, others lockable bags that are great for taking on the go. I've got Stashlogix bags that are fantastic for discretely and conveniently schlepping my stuff around.

Set and setting are critical for having a good experience. Before you get started, think about what you want from the cannabis you're about to consume. Ask yourself how you can get the most benefit from the plant and experience to come. How do you want to use this time and what do you want on hand to make the most of it? Do you want to relax and listen to music or watch TV? Focus and get your to-do list done? Be creative? Be social?

Once you start to feel the effects, you might not be as motivated to get what you want or need. You might forget. It happens! Take care of yourself by taking care of things ahead of time. Be prepared. Have plenty of water or whatever else you want to drink on hand. You may very well get dry mouth. Cottonmouth is a pretty common side effect. Have mints or candies (non-medicated of course) on hand. Healthy snacks available will keep you from going for the stuff you're supposed to avoid, so have them available.

As with most everything else in life, the key to success is to be mindful, release resistance and expectations, and to relax and enjoy the experience. Cannabis is an unbelievable plant with remarkable capabilities to help people heal, find relief and enhance their lives and the world around them. Everyone will develop their own relationship with it and find what works for them. And, ideally, everyone will share their experience with others so that more people will open their minds and can find their own path to healing and well-being.

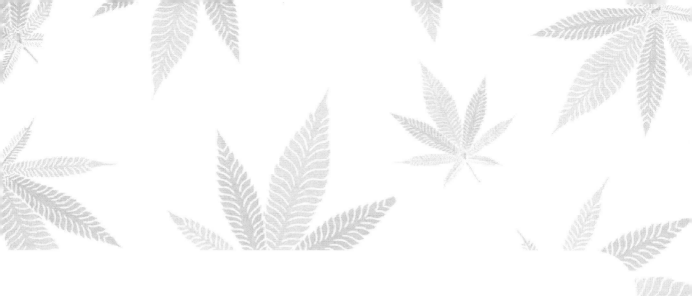

CLOSING QUESTION:

What's the best way to consume cannabis?

There is no best way, there are many ways to enjoy the benefits of weed. It all depends on what you have to consume, where and with whom you're consuming it and what kind of experience you're seeking. Each method has its pros and cons, so what's important is to be conscious and mindful about your consumption: for yourself and for the people around you. Be prepared, so you can have the best experience possible. And most of all, be safe and responsible.

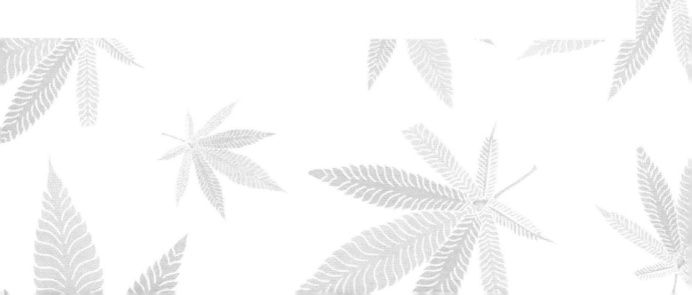

BREAKING THE STIGMA: WORKING WEED INTO YOUR LIFE

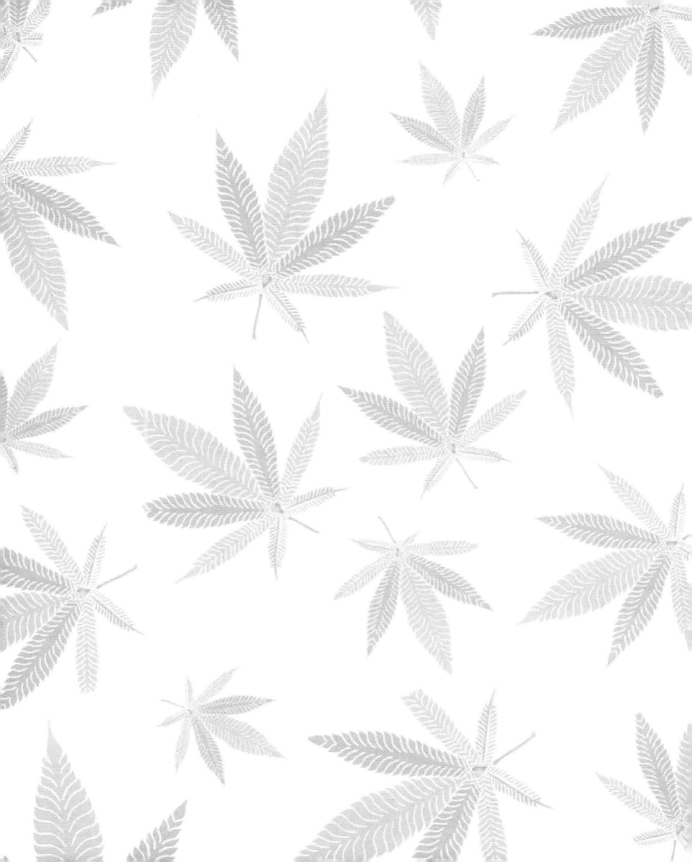

18 COMING OUT OF THE CANNA CLOSET

I hope I've gotten you over long-held misperceptions and fears and you've opened your mind to the possibilities cannabis might offer. Perhaps you've even tried it and realized it's not all that scary or bad after all. You're more comfortable with the idea of marijuana in your body and your life, and so why hide the fact that you've made this choice from the people in your life?

I hear a lot fear about judgment from people—neighbors and friends, physicians, family, whomever. And yes, sometimes even the dog. Far fewer people than you imagine are actually judging you; the fear is in your head for the most part. (The dog is most definitely not judging you. The cat, perhaps…) But yes, there are many who still are unaware, uninformed, closed off or unenlightened. Some will be open to a conversation; some will not. There are ways to test the waters and open the door to a dialogue without exposing yourself.

The Big Reveal: Having the Conversation

When the time is right to have "the talk" with your family or friends, grab this book, take a deep breath (and perhaps a big hit), and pull the ripcord. The key to getting people to talk about cannabis is to actually talk about it.

It might be easiest to start off the discussion with an interesting tidbit about marijuana. Share something surprising you learned in this book. Or share a story you saw about a child who stopped having seizures after taking cannabis oil, or promising research about marijuana stopping Alzheimer's. Refer to the conversation starters (on the opposite page).

Read your audience. If you're getting anger or discomfort, you may want to step back and work on a drip strategy, taking time to share little bits of data and information that can seed a more positive, open-minded dialogue down the road. Otherwise, use the opportunity to take the conversation in a more personal direction. Share your decision (and your experience, if appropriate) in a positive, open way; don't start off defensive and assuming you'll be judged.

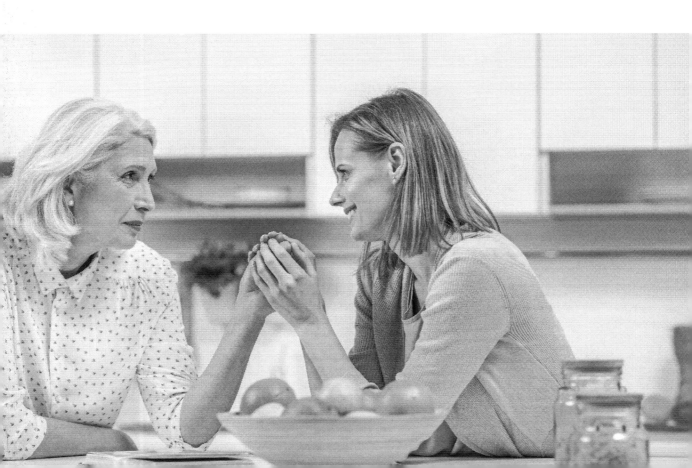

GO ON A FISHING EXPEDITION : IDEAS TO SPARK A DISCUSSION

Here are a few easy ways you can throw a little bait out there to gauge the waters:

Talk about a recent news story or television show you saw about cannabis (a positive one, obvi.) CNN airs re-runs of Dr. Sanjay Gupta's *Weed* series, VICE has a great show called *Weediquette* and there's even a *Shark Tank* for pot entrepreneurs.

Reference an unexpected yet respected person or celebrity who supports weed. Rick Steves, Steven King, Carl Sagan, Maya Angelou, Susan Sarandon and Kathy Bates are all not the traditional face of the cannabis consumer.

Share a story of someone you know benefiting from marijuana (it could even be you!) A personal connection to cannabis can make it seem less foreign and scary; and who doesn't love to hear a success story?

Drop a data point about the tax revenue cannabis is bringing in and how it's being used to benefit children, outdated infrastructures and other worthy beneficiaries. Colorado is bringing in over $10 million *a month* in revenue.

Bring up CBD and what you've learned about its medical benefits. A story or perhaps even an ad could have caught your interest and triggered you to learn more.

Ask if they had any idea that the human body comes with an endocannabinoid system and basically is wired for weed. Most everyone has had a runner's high at some point; it's an easy example to help people understand.

Point out how wrong you were about a marijuana myth, and how surprised you were by the facts. Acknowledging you were wrong could also bring defenses down and help people see they've been fed "alternative facts."

And, if you're hanging out with someone who loves a good conspiracy theory, tell them about the fabricated War on Drugs and history behind Prohibition. That's sure to get a lively conversation started!

Be ready for anything. Awkward silence. Hysteria and tears. Yelling. High fives. A shrug and "good for you." Laughter. Curiosity. You might even hear, "You, too!?" If you've been in the closet, you might find out everyone has known for years. It could lead to an impromptu sesh together, who knows?

There will likely be questions. Some may want to find out more information—perhaps suggest they get themselves a copy of this book! Be patient and give them a chance. Remember there are decades of stigma and misinformation buried deep within most people. Listen to their concerns; in all likelihood, you'll be fully equipped to address each one with an objective counterpoint. (I've given you everything you need to do it.) Let them know you took time to educate yourself and made the decision to consume consciously and intentionally. Share research if you've got it. If you have children at home, address how you'll communicate with them, and how you'll handle your cannabis consumption. If needed, set ground rules about what and when information is shared with the kids. If you're having the conversation with your children, be transparent, consistent and honest; reinforce this is not a license to party and the importance of responsibility and mindfulness.

If you've had a positive experience with cannabis, tell your story and what benefits you've found. If you're using medical marijuana, talk about what symptoms have been relieved and what else you tried before coming to cannabis. Aside from medical benefits, statements like "I find cannabis gives me the ability to stay in the present and helps me stay calm and anxiety-free" are hard to attack. Introduce CBD and the role it plays in today's cannabis world.

Bust a few myths. You're now equipped to counter the go-to myths around marijuana. "But it's addictive! It's a gateway drug! You'll get lung cancer! You'll get fat and lazy!" No, no and no!! Anticipate the concerns and address how you're mitigating them. Cite positive role models—I've given you plenty of names to drop of smart, successful people who are not wasting their lives.

Regardless of where the conversation goes, stay confident and rational. You are not doing anything wrong, not putting anyone at risk and you have no need to apologize or defend your choice. You've made an informed decision, and it's yours to make. That said, if the conversation starts to go off the rails, be willing to drop it. Give time and space for people to digest what you've shared. Come back to the conversation when everyone is more chill.

Don't be disappointed if you don't get a positive response. There are layers of misinformation and misperceptions to unravel; not everyone will be open to a different perspective. Be patient. Let more facts and stories come out organically. Don't force it. But don't be surprised if before long you're laughing about that time you thought the dog was judging you. And who knows? Next Thanksgiving could be puff-puff-pass to Aunt Gail.

By the way, sometimes the conversation doesn't even need to be had. My family, and I know this to be the case for many of my friends, just grew into knowing it. They were in education and reformed hippies, so they certainly were exposed to marijuana. At most I dabbled in college, and I'm sure there was acknowledgement that I'd smoked pot at some point along the way. The "big reveal" for me came when my mom visited me shortly after I'd graduated college—I had a single sprig of a pot plant growing in a cup on the windowsill and didn't bother to hide it. A casual inquiry from her as to when the harvest would be and I no longer was in the closet. (For the record, I have a black thumb and there was no harvest. I'll give you some growing guidance in the next section, but like with rolling joints, it's just not my thing.) It sparked a surprising and enlightening conversation between us.

I found out that my mom, too, had once enjoyed a little pot back in the day. It was the 60s after all. Apparently her sister nearly peed her pants laughing at the cat, but apparently she just got tired and was pretty unimpressed. Plus, she got a job where marijuana was a nonstarter, and those days were done. Over time, my consumption became more open with my family and it was accepted that I used weed. My mom even said she rather I smoke pot than drink, and she was right. It's better for me on all fronts. Flash forward to retirement, and she's starting to open her mind to marijuana and consider how it might make her feel a little less pain, move a little more easily and sleep a little better. Cautiously

MAKE SURE WEED CAN'T BE USED AGAINST YOU

Sadly, not everyone lives in state where cannabis use is legal. And not everyone can engage in a rational, reasonable conversation about cannabis. Even with responsible (and legal) marijuana use, you or someone you love could be subject to persecution. Depending on where you live, the authorities can, and still do, take children from parents if they find marijuana in the home. Tolerance varies from state to state and from town to town. Generally speaking, weed isn't going to be the reason for any involvement from Child Protective Services or the police, but it can be used as a reason to remove kids from parents under the guise of "failure to supervise" or "failure to protect."

Be smart and protect yourself and your family. Foster good relationships. Be dependable. Don't flake out. Don't show up smelling like weed. Do use common sense with an extra serving of awareness and responsibility.

and carefully, and still with skepticism and trepidation she is exploring how cannabis can be used to help her feel and age better. But with each experience and each success story (and with reading this book), she's gaining confidence and seeing more potential in pot, which is my ultimate goal. Oh, and this time around, it was my mom who was paralyzed laughing at the dog and her sister who got tired.

Consuming (or not consuming) cannabis is your choice. And any revelation and conversation about it should also be yours. There are plenty of people who consume discreetly and without any awareness from their family or friends. It is entirely possible. I've given you all the knowledge and tools to consume responsibly and, if need be, on the down low.

But I encourage you to be open and communicative with friends, family and the world at large. (As it makes sense, that is. Weed is still illegal and so I'm not encouraging you to shout from the rooftops or share with the office. Parents with kids at home have Child Protective Services to legitimately fear. Don't put yourself, your family or your job at risk unnecessarily.) This plant works miracles, it simply does. We've been programmed over generations (very intentionally, mind you) to fear marijuana and the fabricated evils that arise from its consumption. There is an outdated system in place that desperately needs to

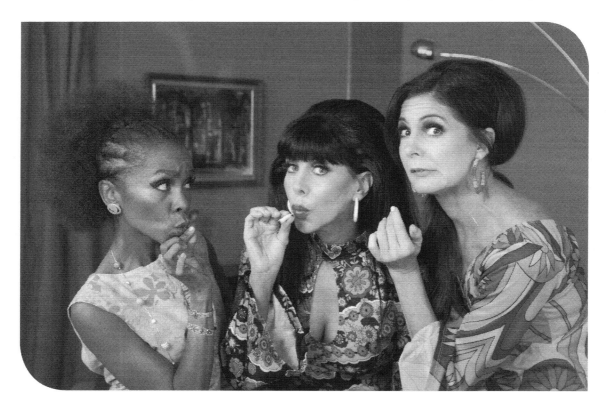

be overhauled; ignorance and false information perpetuate, despite a flood of data coming out in direct conflict with the myths and misperceptions.

The stigma is really sticky. People still judge, even when they're being open-minded. Many are okay with medical marijuana but apply the stoner stereotype to any other consumption (my parents may have been guilty of that until I started writing this book!) I challenge that, and ask you to as well. It is perfectly okay to enjoy cannabis recreationally (responsibly, mindfully and in moderation) without feeling guilty or like you need to justify yourself. Much as people enjoy a little wine at the end of a day or with dinner, a little weed can be a healthier way to unwind. It can bring people closer to together, spark bouts of laughter, inspire and bring a sense of awe and delight. What is wrong with any of this?

Change to the system takes time and moves at a glacial pace. Where real change is going to happen, and will stick, will be with the people. We're waking up to see what cannabis can do to cure diseases, bring health and relief and foster a sense of well-being. We're finding out that it's all been a crock of lies, politics and business interests cooked up to elevate other, self-serving agendas. Our eyes and minds are opening to this plant that has been with us for thousands of years and is natural, harmless and should be readily available to the people who need and want it. What follows will be demand. Consumer demand for safe, consistent products in an ever-expanding number of choices. Public demand for access and legalization. Business demand for the financial and technical infrastructure to support an industry that will be in the hundreds of billions before long.

There are a lot of individuals and far too many businesses and organizations still fighting to keep cannabis in the closet and away from the people who can benefit from it. Whether from a position of ignorance or from one of greed, the war on weed is a losing battle in the long run. No matter what happens at the legislative level, weed isn't going anywhere. It is the next big thing. Those of us who see what weed can do will continue to turn people on to the possibilities cannabis can offer. Show its impact and prove its potential. Build a groundswell of acceptance that will take root and seed future generations with an entirely different perspective of cannabis and the role it plays in our world.

Don't be afraid to open the door and come out of the closet. The monsters aren't real. It's safe. There are a lot of us on the other side of the door, waiting to welcome you to the world of weed, not judge you. You now have the ammunition to counter ignorance and fear. And, by stepping out into the light you might inspire others to come out of the closet, too; or at the very least, to not fear it. Speak up and share that you're in a relationship with cannabis—we do it when we find a person or resource that is amazing. Cannabis deserves your respect and support, too!

Modern Family: the Cannabis Conundrum

For many, the intersection of family and cannabis can create both angst and complexity. We are the sandwich generation, with middle-aged mothers and fathers tending to young adults and older parents, oftentimes living under the same roof.

I am not a parent. I have no direct experience with this subject. But I do know quite a few parents and for the most part, they have been honest and open with their families—of course at the right time and in the proper context. I can't tell you when or if to have "the talk" with your family or how to address the "do as I say, not as I do" with teens and younger children. Every situation and dynamic is unique. I've given you lots of information and facts to support a conversation, framed to support whatever benefits you receive from marijuana.

But I can advise that in any healthy relationship, transparency and honesty are critical. Like the sex talk, it may be uncomfortable and awkward, but your kids will appreciate it. Equally important is open dialogue, so give space for your family to have concerns or set boundaries in terms of what is okay to discuss and when it is okay (or not okay) to consume in front of the young'uns.

When all is said and done, only you can know if and when the time is right to come out of the closet. I can't tell you what's right for your family and how cannabis should be handled. But, I will reinforce to you that, no matter open and transparent you are with kids about consumption, you need to keep your cannabis safe and securely stored out of the reach of tiny humans.

On Pot and (Grand)Parenting

Thankfully we are seeing less of the knee-jerk reactions of horror from people when the topic of cannabis and children comes up. News stories about kids who stop having debilitating seizures after just a tiny dose of cannabis oil proliferate. The Today Show is airing segments on cannabis dinners and marijuana moms. Brave and bold mothers have spoken up and spoken out to help break the stigma and misperception, and have gone to the limits to get medicine for their children in need.

We are making progress, but many of the same people who judge someone for choosing to consume cannabis think nothing of knocking back a couple of glasses of wine or a cocktail. In front of their children, to boot! And how many people are walking around zonked out on pharmaceuticals while functioning in their daily lives?

So, let's come back to common sense. Conscious, responsible consumption does not put children at risk. In fact, for many people it makes them better (grand)parents and better able to enjoy family bonding experiences. If you feel better, whatever "better" means for you, you can be more engaged, more present and even perhaps more patient.

Speaking of patience, let me address the shadow side of the pot and parenting conversation: Pot should never be used as a coping tool. Much like you shouldn't be downing a bottle of chardonnay to get through the night, you shouldn't be using weed to check out and disengage with your family.

Medical Marijuana for Kids?

To reiterate: I am not a doctor, nor do I play one on TV. I cannot advise whether medical marijuana is right for your (grand)child or someone you love. That is a decision to be made after much more research and discussion with family and physicians. What I can say with confidence is that there are children, many of them, who have found relief in medical marijuana when all other efforts have failed. Turn on the TV or turn to the internet and you'll see tragic stories of children fighting devastating illness who have been given a lifeline in the form of cannabis.

The coverage started with Charlotte Figi, the young girl who suffered from hundreds of grand mal seizures a week; with cannabis therapy, little Charlotte now only suffers from seizures on occasion. Kids with cancer and a host of other conditions are feeling and often getting better with the help of cannabis. Parents are seeing their children go from debilitatingly sick to happy and healthy. They're stepping up their activism, and politicians are starting to respond. They're pushing physicians for alternative therapies and access to natural medicine, driving doctors to consider a broader perspective and toolset in treating their patients.

While healthy kids should not be consuming cannabis; children suffering from a host of illnesses and conditions can and do benefit from medical marijuana. Whether that decision is right for your family can only be made by your family and the professionals who work with you to help keep your family healthy and whole.

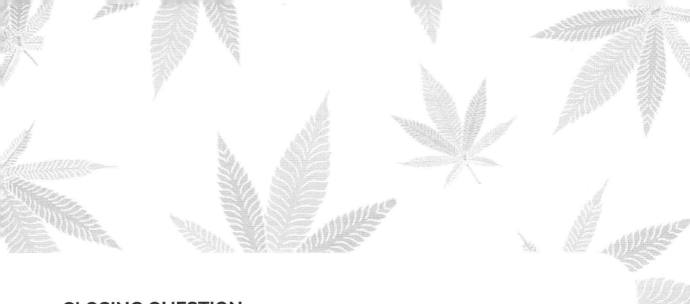

CLOSING QUESTION:

How do I have the conversation about cannabis?

It might be easier than you think, but even if it's difficult, it's best to be honest and open with the people you feel should know about cannabis and whatever thoughts or experience you have with it. There are plenty of opportunities to spark a common sense conversation about weed and ways to open the door to a deeper discussion about cannabis, its benefits and responsible consumption. And if I might point out, you now have this book. Perhaps you should suggest it as reading!

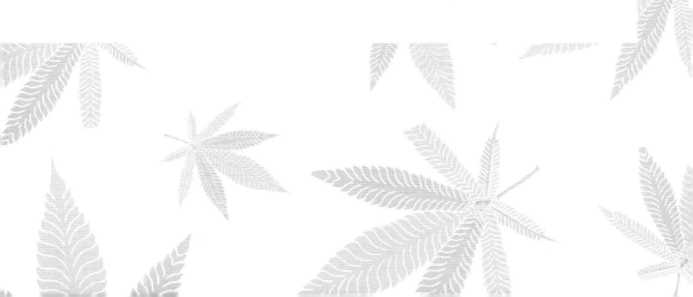

19 WAYS IN WHICH WEED CAN MAKE YOUR LIFE BETTER

I'm betting a good majority of Baby Boomers and younger retirees tried weed way back in the day, but then grew up and started to care about things like illegality and stigma. With the crumbling of those barriers, more and more people are coming back to it; or at least are thinking about it!

Beyond the potential medical and therapeutic benefits of marijuana, there is broader application to help an aging population age better. Physiological benefits that help our skin and joints. Health and wellness benefits that help enhance and connect body, mind and spirit. Life enrichment benefits that help us engage with and enjoy the activities and people that make a full and rewarding life. No matter how you look at it, when it comes to overall health and wellness, cannabis can help aging brains and bodies function better, and add a little pixie dust to your life as well!

Going Green in Your Golden Years: Aging Well

For anyone concerned with aging well, pay attention: weed is good for an aging body and mind. I repeat, weed is good for us as we age.

Beyond the ways in which cannabis combats disease, illness and a host of other conditions, weed is uniquely able to tap into our bodies' own regulatory system to fight the ravages of aging. Poor diet, chronic stress, prevalence of toxic chemicals and lack of exercise all throw our system out of balance. Everything that comes with getting older can be attributed to inflammation and the effects of free radicals. And guess what? Cannabis can give the body a boost to fight disease and the effects of aging. Cannabinoids are potent antioxidants that can neutralize wrinkles as well as cancer-causing free radicals. Can you think of anything else that can do both?

Remember, your endocannabinoid system (ECS) regulates everything in your body. It's the key to homeostasis, balance and a smoothly running system. It can slow the signs of aging and fight a host of age-related illnesses. Your ECS doesn't just protect your insides; since our skin is our largest organ, it has lots of endocannabinoid receptors that, when activated, can fight free radicals and other stuff that causes us to age. These receptors can also reduce itching and irritating skin issues like psoriasis and eczema. Cannabis is uniquely able to tap into our endocannabinoid system. How about that?

Our skin is our first line of defense against various environmental stressors and pathogens, and carries the most visible signs of aging, especially when exposed to years of stress and sun damage. As we age, the body's skin becomes dry, loses elasticity and even loses some of its ability to heal itself from different infections, skin diseases and viruses. Lipid production goes down and eventually stops. Fortunately, cannabis can protect aging skin and even treat skin diseases; and even hemp oil, the legal way to weed, contains a variety of antioxidants and is rich in essential Omega-3 and Omega-6 fatty acids.

Beyond the skin, cannabis goes to work in the brain and body. On a molecular level, cannabinoids help regulate energy production, acting as antioxidants and essentially giving your body an oxygen cleanse. This increases brain activity and destroys free radicals in the process.

Weed even helps an aging brain. We've already talked about the promise THC is showing in battling Alzheimer's and dementia. But do you know what else it may do? Reverse aging and improve memory in older brains. Yup, once again, it seems weed actually is good for your brain. Scientists say that THC is showing early signs of slowing down and even reversing the aging process in mice: low-dose THC given to aging mice boosted their performance on cognitive tasks. In fact the performance of elderly mice matched that of mice in their prime. Dad (and all you other competitors out there), are you listening? By the way, those same tests were done on younger mice and guess what? Cognition worsened. Just like with young humans. (We're talking tests on mice, so don't get carried away yet!)

Bones and joints are also pain points, quite literally, for most of us as we age. Cannabis reduces inflammation and swelling, in addition to relieving pain, for osteoarthritis and rheumatoid arthritis sufferers. And guess what? When you don't ache and creak, all of a sudden you feel a lot younger. All those cannabinoids also help broken bones heal faster and protect against osteoporosis, so that if you do suffer from a fall or weakening bones, cannabis can speed healing and slow bone degradation.

A LITTLE GANJA A DAY...

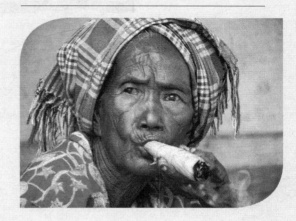

Fulla Nayak, the world's oldest woman, was 125 years old when she passed away in 2006 in India. She attributed her longevity to smoking marijuana every day (and drinking a little wine)!

And don't forget I told you about weed's potential ability to keep people thinner and have lower blood sugar, as well as to bring blood pressure down. Pot truly is a potent and powerful preventative health tool when you think about it.

Weed, Fitness and Well-Being
(Yes, You Can Get Off the Couch!)

Despite the couch-potato stigma that comes with stoner stereotypes, there are plenty of people who consume cannabis and are healthy, fit and active. Studies are showing weed seems to boost metabolism, speed fat loss and lower blood sugar and cholesterol. We all know the importance of exercise and wellness in maintaining optimum health and keeping the extra pounds at bay. If you'll recall your lesson on the endocannabinoid system (ECS), that runner's high we get when endorphins are released with a good workout is pretty much the same as a marijuana high. Exercise activates the endocannabinoid system in the same way that cannabis does. That feeling is what keeps many of us coming back. And to be clear, no, I'm not saying you can swap weed for a good workout; but the two do go well together.

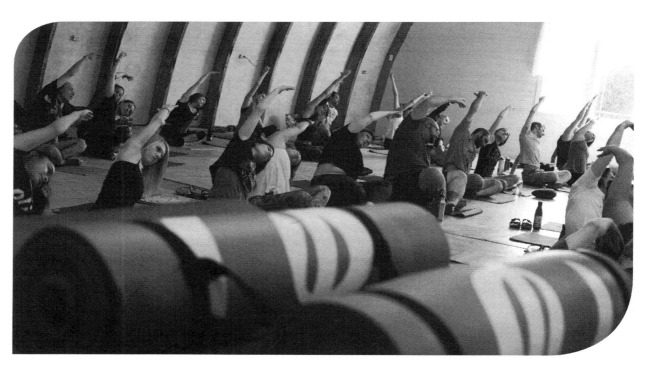

Mason Jar Event Group's Yoga With a View

I am not one of those people who loves to exercise. This has nothing to do with the weed, it's been a lifelong challenge for me. But I do enjoy feeling strong and healthy, and have found yoga and meditation to be my way to health and wellness. And with a gym in my building, I do force myself to get onto the elliptical machine on occasion. For me, a few hits on the vape pen before I go to a class or hit the elliptical helps me stay focused and present, and perhaps more beneficially, keeps me from getting antsy and looking at the clock every five minutes. I can relax more deeply into my poses. I'm not running through my to-do's or chasing thought bubbles.

For those who do love to exercise, you might be interested to know that an increasing number of athletes are turning to marijuana as a training tool. Remember that lung capacity and breathing actually improve with smoking (or vaping) cannabis. (It clearly didn't take anything away from Michael Phelps performance!) Pain thresholds are higher, which can help you push through barriers to progress. It goes without saying this can work to your disadvantage; you may feel less pain, but it's there for a reason. Chances are you're not going pro, so always tune in and listen to your body. If you do push it a bit too far, a cannabis topical can ease aching muscles and joints.

MARIJUANA AND MASSAGE

Cannabis topicals can make a delightful and revitalizing addition to a spa treatment or pampering massage. (Yes, there are 420-friendly spas and therapists in legal states.) Infused oils, lotions, bath salts and balms can all help tight muscles loosen up and unwind…I would categorize that as "wellness!"

With more 420-friendly fitness options becoming available in legal states, it can actually be fun to hit the vape and then hit the class! Working out doesn't have to be a grind, make it something you might actually enjoy.

As with everything, find what works for you in a safe and conscious way. You don't want to try yoga for the first time in years if you're a little wobbly after a little weed. Start with taking the dog for a light hike or long walk. Try your vape pen when you're going to be on an exercise bike or something with handles. If you can find a 420 class or gym, talk to a trainer about safe ways to bring cannabis into your routine (or to spark a new routine, if you need something new and different to get you moving).

Beyond the physical benefits, marijuana helps you get into the flow. Or zone. Or whatever you want to call it. But it's that place where anxiety disappears, focus increases and awareness is enhanced. This can help you power through your 25 minutes on the stairmaster or 26 miles of a marathon (or a PowerPoint presentation, or a power cleaning of your house. You get the idea. Flow state is real and a fantastic place to be).

Could Pot Be the Key to a Happier Life?

We live in a world of to-do lists, juggling responsibilities, work-hard-to-get-ahead mentality and a (faulty) belief that success requires always setting goals, getting it done and then moving on to the next thing as quickly as possible. Many of us get so caught up in the pursuit of accomplishment and getting things done that we don't stop to be happy, grateful and fulfilled in the moment. The chase of what we think will make us happy becomes more of the focus than actually enjoying what does make us happy. And, happiness doesn't just happen once a box gets checked.

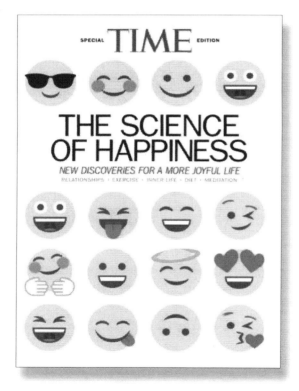

Science is showing us that slowing down and being present, instead of running through your to-do list and thinking about what's next, makes you more successful on all fronts. You're more productive. Less anxious. Happier. And it gives you charisma apparently! When we are in tune with and focused on what we're doing, we enjoy it more fully and become absorbed and engaged.

Cutting-edge research recently published in a special edition from *TIME* shows us that there is a direct relationship between happiness and health: "The Science of Happiness" brings real science to the old cliché, "don't worry, be happy." Sadly we only spend about half our time in the present moment—but when we do, we are at our happiest, no matter what we're doing. This goes for stuff we don't like doing as well, so if you're stuck with a chore or project you hate, don't start thinking about what else you'd rather be doing. Embrace the suck and power through it with presence.

When you're present, you fully experience what is going on around you. You slow down and are actually with the people you're with, immersed in what you're doing or discussing and are engaged and connected. Not only will you be happier and more productive, the people around you will appreciate your presence and attention—and better relationships generally beget success and happiness. How about that?

For many, cannabis can be a powerful tool for presence and grounding. And don't forget one of the more straightforward benefits of marijuana: everything is better on weed. If one path to happiness is to truly experience pleasure, to be fully into the feeling and the experience, then weed will happily lead you down that path. Savoring the sensation of touch or a burst of flavors in your mouth is taken to new heights of bliss and enjoyment with a little weed floating around your system.

Marijuana and mindfulness go hand in hand. It can tame your monkey brain and bring you into the present; ease your mind and your body so you can be fully in the moment. Pot can make meditation easier and even open up a whole new inner world. It can even help with breathing (I know, you're still having a hard time buying the whole weed-is-good-for-your-lungs idea.) This is all with the right strain, of course; the wrong one will send you in the opposite direction of centered and focused. Weed is not one-size-fits-all, as we've already covered!

If spirituality is your thing, it can help you connect more deeply to spirit, nature and earth, expand your consciousness and take you into higher vibrations of love and light. Plants can offer wisdom and healing; some believe they have the ability to communicate with each other and with us, and can connect us to spiritual realms. Cannabis has been used for thousands of years by ancient and indigenous peoples in religious and spiritual ceremonies and practices; it can be sacred and powerful plant medicine.

Microdosing as a Daily Wellness Regimen

Perhaps one of the hottest topics in cannabis these days is microdosing: the technique of taking only small quantities of substances for therapeutic purposes. In case you haven't heard, more and more people (particularly high-performing professionals and creative folks) are doing it to enhance productivity and inspiration, as well as treat various mental-health conditions such as depression, anxiety, PTSD and ADHD. You might still see video clips on TV or social media of all the kids dabbing, but people are talking about the therapeutic benefits of microdosing.

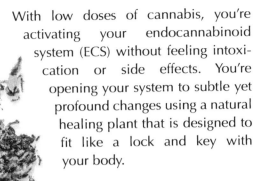

With low doses of cannabis, you're activating your endocannabinoid system (ECS) without feeling intoxication or side effects. You're opening your system to subtle yet profound changes using a natural healing plant that is designed to fit like a lock and key with your body.

If you're prone to anxiety on cannabis, don't like how it makes you feel, want to be more focused and relaxed or want to drop the meds you're taking—microdosing might be for you.

As I've reinforced throughout the book, take it low and slow, and be mindful and aware as to how you feel and how your body is responding. Slow and steady is the goal here. Every body is different, dosing is not one-size-fits-all; and even your own physiology will change from day to day based on body chemistry, moods and other factors. You will also build up a tolerance over time, so adjusting dosing or spacing out timing can keep you at your desired level.

If you're using edibles to microdose, the range is generally 1–5 mg. You can also take a puff or two on a vaporizer; the key is not to actually feel any overt effects. Pay attention to the potency and cannabinoid profile of what you're consuming, and go for a 1:1 CBD/THC ratio if possible.

What you get from microdosing will vary depending on what you're consuming. You may feel a bit more relaxed, more energetic or more focused. You may find more creativity, presence and heightened awareness. You can use it to relieve stress and ease pain and reduce the chronic inflammation we all face without having to worry about intense psychoactivity. Microdosing can be great for medicating while working or taking care of the family.

Invite Mary Jane Over for Sexy Time!

Cannabis under the covers can take sex to new highs. I mean, it doesn't turn you into a sex-crazed maniac and lead to drug-fueled orgies. It certainly doesn't lead to drug-crazed abandon. But it just might unleash your passions. Most people who enjoy a little weed before getting busy find it enhances the experience. I personally give it two thumbs up (sorry, mom and dad)!

It shouldn't be surprising, if you've been following along so far. Cannabis relaxes muscles, and can ease anxiety and enhance your mood. It can make you feel euphoric. When you're relaxed, it's easier to lower inhibitions. It can heighten sensation, boost the intensity of your pleasure and even make it easier to have the big "O." There are even products specifically designed to enhance intimacy and pleasure—you'd be surprised at what a little weed can do for you! Brands like Foria are gaining popularity as people find new, fun ways that cannabis can enhance experiences, in addition to relief and relaxation.

Stressed out? Unwind together with an indica or hybrid that has myrcene in its profile. Or enjoy a sensuous massage with cannabis

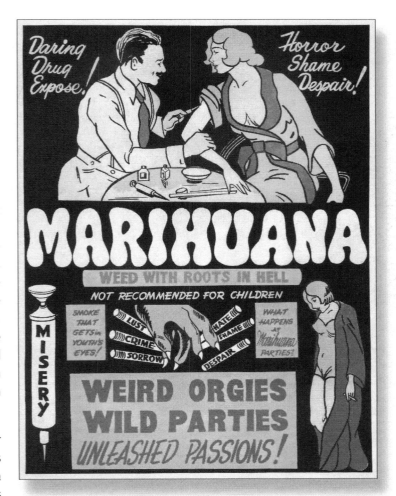

or hemp oil. Want to add a little spark and energy to bring some sizzle into the sheets? Try a sativa rich in limonene. By the way, there are now products like weed lube and sensual enhancement oils to bring new sensations to your nether regions. They won't get you high, but they just might help you get off.

A few words of advice, just to keep things safe and pleasurable:

- Don't get too high! Relaxed and happy is good; drooling and dopey is not. You want to be able to function and to be connected to your experience and to your partner, not checked out. Too much weed won't affect performance like too much alcohol will, but it can still take you out of your passion zone. I've given you all the guidance you need to keep your consumption in check. The rest is up to you!

- Do test the waters. If you're trying something (or someone) new, you want an idea of how it's going to make you feel. The last thing you want is to feel dizzy or paranoid.

- Do be ready for dryness. I've warned you that cottonmouth can be a side effect of weed—what is normally an inconvenience can become interference with a dry mouth. Have plenty of water within reach. Mints or hard candies are also good to have around. And it works the same down there for us ladies. Have some lube on hand, in case you need a little helping hand.

> ## IS WEED AN APHRODISIAC?
>
> Not exactly. It's not a sexual stimulant per se, but it does enhance the sensory and sensual experience. In this case, the expression "Everything's better with weed" is (G) spot on!

- Don't smoke in bed, particularly after you've done the deed. Whether you're dozing or diddling, you could be distracted and end up ruining your bedding, or worse yet, setting you or your partner on fire. You want smoking hot sex, not a smoking hot bed.

Make Your Second Childhood Even Better Than the First!

Assuming you have more free time on your hands once young kids no longer require constant attention, supervision and shuttling around, there's a world of possibility to explore. Travel, hobbies, learning, creating, socializing, playing, entertaining, reconnecting with friends and loved ones, reconnecting with yourself and the world around you...all are activities that can be enhanced through conscious consumption of cannabis.

Beyond the vast range of medical benefits, weed can help tap into long-buried playfulness, creativity and joy. It can help spark a second childhood, where you feel wonder and awe, and giggle until your sides hurt. Where you learn new things, create and explore. Play for the fun of it. Lose track of time. Take time to watch the clouds. That is what life is about after all. We're not put here to just work or be serious all the time. We're here to have experiences and make connections, to create whatever is our heart's desire.

A painting class that helps you spark your creativity and inspiration? A dinner party with cannabis pairings that rival the finest wine tasting? Yoga and meditation with extra presence and relaxation? A few hits from the vape pen on the golf course to relax and loosen up? Bridge club can be taken to a whole new level. A light hike can take on extra beauty and bring added awe. Anything is possible.

Around the country more and more businesses are cropping up to cater to the canna-consumer and offer curated experiences. There are events (and event-planning services) that bring conscious cannabis consumption into the mix—these are not wild club parties. We're talking elegant dinners, yoga classes and retreats, singles mixers, cannabis tasting parties and more. Spas offer cannabis-infused treatments. You can take painting and writing classes, or learn how to cook with cannabis. There are even gyms and fitness classes where you can bend, blaze and bulk up. Travel companies have canna-packages. Bud & breakfasts are sprouting and consumption-friendly transportation will get you to where you're going while taking you around town.

Use the interweb to find local classes, resources and events; or look for a cannabis-specific event calendar for goings-on in your area. As cannabis comes out of the closet, you'll find more and more options to integrate a little weed into your life, if that's your jam.

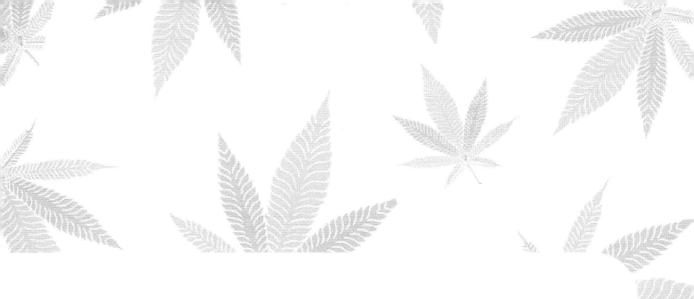

CLOSING QUESTION:

Are you kidding, weed helps with wrinkles and wellness?

I can't tell you that cannabis is the next big beauty secret (someone will, just not me!)—but I can say with confidence that weed helps brains and bodies age better. It can help you find the zone in a workout; bring gratitude and presence (keys to a happy life it seems!); ease stress and enhance relationships; and experience the joy in simply enjoying life and enriching yourself through a range of activities. We work hard our entire lives to get to this point: why not enjoy it to the highest potential?

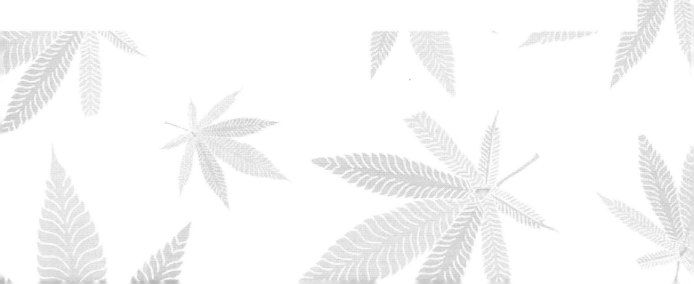

20 GET COOKING IN THE KITCHEN AND ELEVATE ANY CUISINE

One of cannabis' greatest gifts is her ability to enhance just about any experience. Food tastes better. Music moves you in new ways. The world around you is brighter. Scents smell amazing. Activities are more fun. Crowds are less annoying. Whatever it is you're doing, it's better on weed.

As cannabis comes out of the closet, we get to experiment and explore the many ways it can be incorporated into both everyday life and special celebrations. From daily edibles microdosing to weed weddings, there's no limit—beyond legalities of course—to bringing cannabis into your life, if you choose to do so.

Before you start infusing marijuana into pretty much whatever your heart desires, be sure you have plenty of non-medicated food around to supplement whatever you're preparing. Whether as part of a multi-course meal or a single delightful bite, you always want to be able to satisfy the desire for "more" with food that is both safe and tasty.

MAKE READY FOR THE MUNCHIES!

While not a given, there is a good chance you'll get the munchies along the way. Weed doesn't just make you want to eat; it makes everything taste better. This can go for the new flavor of Doritos or a luxe meal; your tongue is going to be happy no matter what you put on it. If you're going to be at home, be prepared and have on hand whatever food will pleasure your palate. I suggest giving yourself options for savory and sweet, and refrain from cooking anything. Keep it simple, nourishing and delicious and you won't go wrong (or kill your waistline). Oh, and definitely don't go shopping while you're high—it will be a costly trip. I know all too well.

Stir it Up: Cooking With Cannabis

Making your own edibles opens up a world of canna-cuisine, whether you're a fan of Top Chef or Chef Boyardee. It can be as simple as adding a drop or two of activated concentrate or tincture; or you can incorporate an infused butter or oil into elevated haute cuisine. Generally speaking, you don't want to just grind up some weed and throw it into your food; it will be gross, and unless you've put the appropriate heat to it, it won't be activated (remember that THC doesn't become psychoactive until it's decarboxylated.) It's possible to work finely ground bud into things like meatballs and strongly flavored sauces, but unless the flavor is strong enough to cover the weed, there are far better ways for tasty and effective cannabis consumption.

Home cooking also gives you the advantage of choice, control and customization. Oh, and it's cheaper, too! While you can find this with commercial edibles in some markets and with some brands, the vast majority of options are sugary treats

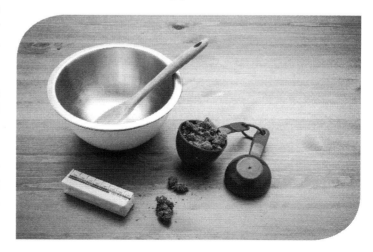

and not savory, healthy fare (which apparently doesn't sell). Beyond giving yourself more options to please your palate, making your own edibles lets you control the strain and customize the dosing. It's always good to know what you're going to get, but this is particularly beneficial to a medical marijuana patient. Remember how different strains are good for different conditions? You can choose the strains that will deliver the cannabinoid profiles targeted for whatever ails you.

The foundation for any infused cooking is cannabutter or oil. Once you've got that, you can create just about any food you fancy. Once it's made, using it is no different than using non-medicated cooking fat. Think beyond brownies and cookies. Salad dressing. Oatmeal. I am sought after (and award-winning) for my medicated mac & cheese. Read on; I'll share my recipe!

Making cannabutter or oil can take a little time and patience, but is relatively simple. Cannabis needs to be heated at low temperatures over long periods of time. As with eating it, with cooking it's "low and slow." You can do this on the stove or in a crockpot. The key is that you don't want it to get too hot too quickly and burn off all those good cannabinoids.

By the way, if infusing foods at home is something you plan to do with any frequency, you might want to pick up a device designed specifically for making cannabutter and oil. It makes things much simpler and cleaner (which is what kitchen appliances are supposed to do, eh?) Some of the newest models, like the one I have from LEVO Oil, are gorgeous, and look like any other device on your counter. And you can also use it to infuse herbs and other deliciousness into other oils and butters, giving you both versatility and legitimacy when your mother-in-law (or daughter-in-law) asks you what kind of coffeemaker you bought. Of course, you can also use that as an opportunity to start a conversation…just sayin'.

FOR A BASIC CALCULATION:

Assume 1 stick of butter = 7 grams of weed (¼ ounce) = 700 mg of THC.

Guidance for dosing per serving

Beginner: 5–10 mg

Experienced: 20–30 mg

Heavy: 40–60 mg

Making Cannabutter or Oil

You can make your infusion with anything from leaves and trim to the biggest buds; it depends on what you have on hand and what you want to spend. Home growers tend to use trim to make the most use of the plant; people who are buying it tend to cook with lower-quality shake or bud to keep things more economical. For canna-connoisseurs without limitations or growers with an abundance of flower, cooking with high-quality bud bring the A-game to the kitchen. Foodies and cannophiles are matching terpene profiles of cannabis to flavor profiles of foods to create elevated dining experiences that push the boundaries of creativity and cuisine.

What goes into the mix will drive how much to use. Higher quality cannabis generally means you need less of it. Strain profiles and potency will also influence what kind of concoction you create to deliver the desired effects. You're using dried plant material, by the way, not fresh green leaves or buds.

HOW MUCH WEED SHOULD I USE?

Ratios will differ depending on how strong or light you want the butter to be, how potent the marijuana is and the cannabis-to-fat ratio you want. The foundational recipe is one ounce of weed for four sticks of butter (and therefore, you'd use a half ounce for two sticks of butter.) If you're a newbie, start with a half-ounce of weed to four sticks of butter, gradually increasing the cannabis until you're familiar with the results. Microdosers will want far less. Remember that you'll need more trim or shake than bud to achieve the same potency.

To estimate the total dosage for your batch of butter or oil, you have to calculate THC/gram and then multiply that by how many grams you're using. For average weed, assume 100 mg of THC per gram; for the high-grade stuff, use 150 mg/gram. For example: 7 grams of average weed (¼ ounce) would give you 700 mg of THC.

If you're looking to keep the potency low per serving, you can use a few tactics beyond simply making a less potent infusion. You can make more servings out of your batch to up the recipe yield. Choose a recipe that doesn't use a lot of fat in it—for example rice krispie treats take less butter than a brownie recipe. Or simply use less of the fat in whatever you're making and mix it with a non-medicated version.

Making Your Cannabutter on the Stovetop or Slow Cooker

First, prepare your workspace and gather up your materials. You should have already calculated how much butter and weed you're using. You will need:

Weed (ground finely with seeds and stems removed)

Butter

Medium saucepan or a slow cooker

Cheesecloth

Water

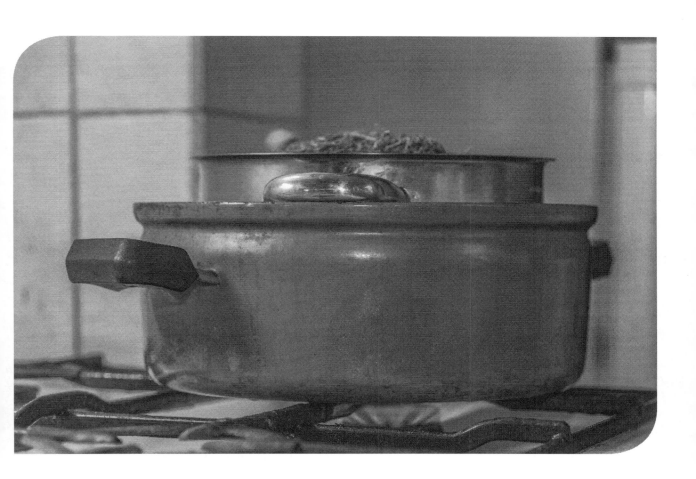

1 **DECARB YOUR CANNABIS:** Heat oven to 240 degrees. Spread the weed in a single layer on a baking sheet (with sides). Bake for 40 minutes, turning the sheet a couple of times to ensure even heating. The cannabis will become dry and crumbly. This is not a must-do, but for those seeking maximum potency, it's worth the extra step.

2 **SIMMER:** If making on the stovetop, combine 4 cups of water, butter (cut into several pieces) and ground cannabis into a medium saucepan and cook over low heat—the mixture should never boil but simply simmer. (You can also use a double boiler.) Stir every 30 minutes or so and continue cooking for 3–4 hours. The mixture will thicken up, but don't let it get too thick or let the cannabis touch the bottom of the pan; if needed, add a bit more water. It's done when the top of the mix turns from really watery to glossy and thick. Turn off heat and allow to cool.

If you're using a slow cooker, combine butter, weed and water and cook on low for 6 to 10 hours. You can let it go longer if you choose. The longer you let it simmer the richer it becomes in terpenes. And you know those terps are influential little suckers.

3 **STRAIN:** Line a colander or strainer with a double layer of cheesecloth (make sure it overhangs or secure it). When cool enough to handle, pour the mixture into the cheesecloth—make sure you have a bowl or container to catch all the butter. Press down with a spatula to get the butter through, leaving behind the plant material. Gather up the cheesecloth and twist tightly to squeeze out the remaining butter. When you've gotten it all out, toss the cheesecloth.

4 **COOL & PREP:** Place in the fridge until the butter has solidified and risen to the top layer. Run a knife around the edge and lift the butter off. Place upside down on a work surface and scrape off any of the cooking water. Your butter will be green. Do not be alarmed. Place in an airtight container and refrigerate until ready to use.

Cannabutter can be stored in the fridge for up to two months and retain its potency.

To make infused oil, the same principles apply. Low and slow. Oil is much more prone to scorching, so never let it get over 245 degrees. Determine which oil you want to use: canola, olive and coconut are all good options, but anything will work. Note that oils with a higher fat content absorb the most THC from the plant. Use one ounce of weed to two cups of oil as the foundation.

Get Eating!
Recipes & Recommendations to Get You Started

There's a world of canna-cuisine to explore. There's really no limit to what you can medicate and enjoy. Before you get started, here are a few pro tips to help you stave off failure and get the most from the infusion you've just created.

- Direct high heat can damage cannabinoids, so temperature management is key. Never heat above 392 degrees (F.) Whenever possible, as with dosing and making the actual infusion, "low and slow" is better.

- Use cannabutter for baking, rather than frying.

- Never go above medium heat; don't fry or saute with infused oils.

- Don't use infused oils for marinades; very little actually gets absorbed into the food and you've wasted all those good cannabinoids. Salad dressings and things you actually swallow are the way to go.

- Your infusion is going to be herbacious; depending on how much weed you used, it could get pretty weedy (and green!). Season appropriately to hide or bring out the flavor in your cannabutter or oil. Extracts, spices and flavorings can be a good canna-chef's secret weapon.

Don't forget that you can take any recipe and add a small amount of activated cannabis concentrate (like a CO_2 oil or RSO oil) or tincture to make an instant edible. It's just drop and go.

Assuming you have your infused butter or oil, here are a few of my favorite recipes to help spark ideas for your culinary exploration. The sky's the limit—have fun getting your Julia Child on!

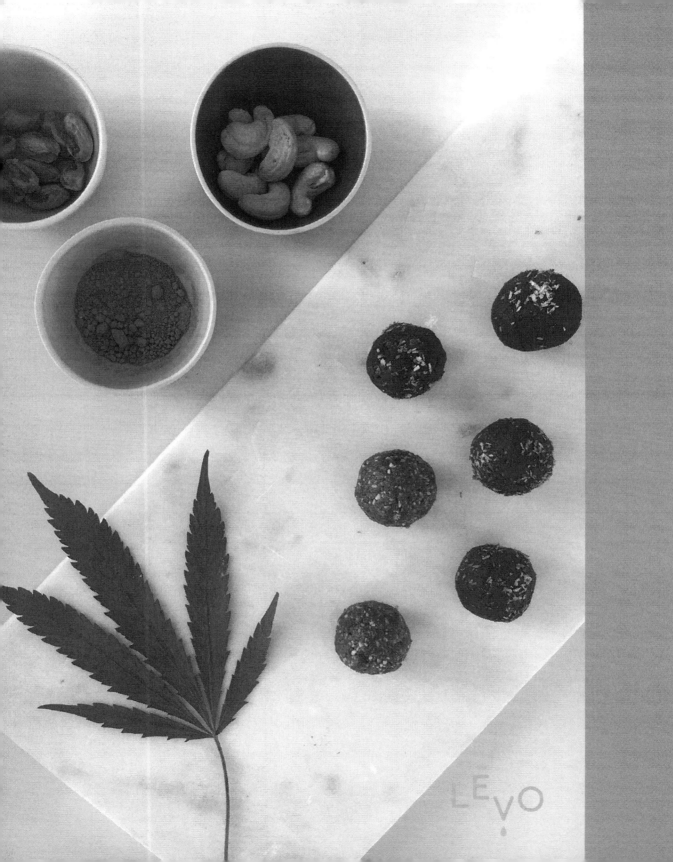

PISTACHIO MATCHA SNACK BALLS
Delicious mircrodosed nibbles, courtesy of my friends at LEVO Oil!

Ingredients:

1 ½ c raw cashews

1 ½ c raw pistachio nuts

1 ½ c medjool dates, pitted

2 tsp matcha powder

1 tbsp infused coconut oil

¼ tsp ground cardamom

1 tbsp grated lemon rind

2 tbsp desiccated coconut

¼ tsp salt

Raw cacao powder for dusting

Instructions:

Combine all ingredients in a food processor and blend until mixture resembles wet sand.

Roll mixture into balls, roughly 1 tbsp each

Dust with cacao powder, extra coconut, more matcha or whatever else you fancy!

"WHAT'S YOUR SECRET INGREDIENT?" MAC & CHEESE

You can mix up the cheese in this recipe to your taste—I prefer sharp cheeses with strong flavors and stick to white or light-colored cheese, but this recipe is adaptable and forgiving. Use any combination of cheeses, add-ins (bacon *and* weed make everything better!) and spices to create a tasty fan favorite. You can medicate the mac & cheese itself, or keep it to the topping (and even serve separately) for a lighter and more controllable experience.

Ingredients:

1 lb celletani (or other spiral-like pasta)

8–10 oz. extra sharp cheddar cheese, shredded/grated

8–10 oz. pecorino romano cheese, shredded/grated

8–10 oz. gruyere cheese, shredded/grated

1 c parmesan cheese, shredded/grated

1 clove garlic

4 tbsp infused butter

4 tbsp flour

2 cups milk

½ c sherry (or dry white wine)

¼ tsp nutmeg

½ tsp paprika

½ tsp dry mustard

Salt & pepper to taste

Breadcrumbs (or panko) + parmesan + infused butter for topping

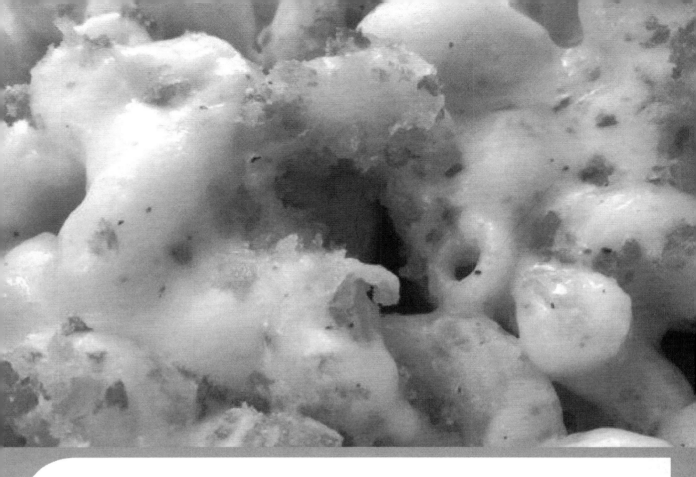

Instructions:

Cook the pasta al dente. While it's cooking, melt butter over very low heat. When melted, whisk in flour (1 tbsp at a time) to make a roux. When smooth, add sherry and whisk until roux is dissolved. Turn up heat to medium-low, add milk and stir frequently until sauce thickens (about 5-7 minutes). While thickening, add spices and adjust to taste.

Add garlic and cheese (a handful or so at a time) and stir until melted. (Hint: I used a food processor to shred the cheese and it was super easy. You can also use small chunks, but the cheese becomes more difficult to melt evenly). When cheese is melted, mix in the pasta and stir well. Pour into buttered casserole/baking dish (I use 9x13 pan).

Melt a little butter and mix with breadcrumbs and parmesan. Sprinkle over the top of the mac & cheese and bake at 350 degrees for approximately 30 minutes or until the top is golden and bubbly.

CHOCOLATE CUPCAKES WITH BACON MAPLE BUTTERCREAM FROSTING

Perfect for game day or really any occasion, these delicious treats take a little extra time and love, but are a flavor explosion of bacon-y delight. I recommend making mini-cupcakes instead of full-sized versions, making it easier to eat, share and manage dosing!

Ingredients:

12 oz package thick cut applewood smoked bacon (plus all the drippings!)

½ cup (or more) maple syrup

1 package devil's food chocolate cake mix

1 box instant chocolate pudding mix

1 cup sour cream

½ cup water

½ cup vegetable oil

4 large eggs

2 sticks infused butter; room temperature

2 teaspoons pure vanilla extract

1 pound confectioners' sugar

1 teaspoon salt

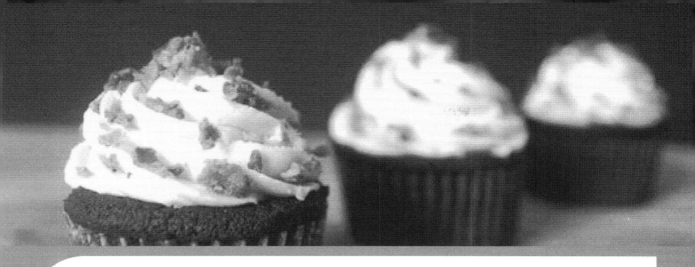

Instructions:

Preheat oven to 350. Grease cupcake pans. Dust with flour and tap out the excess; set pans aside.

First, candy the bacon. Rub bacon with maple syrup, coating it well. (You can also add cayenne or use brown sugar.) Place on a broiler pan with tin foil in the bottom to catch the grease. Bake for 20-25 minutes. Be sure to save the bacon grease! Put bacon aside and blot with paper towels. Once it's cooled and crisped up, chop into small pieces.

Then, make the cupcakes. Place the cake mix, pudding mix, sour cream, water, oil, and eggs in a large mixing bowl. Add about half the bacon grease, reserving 2-3 tbsp for the frosting. Blend with an electric mixer on low speed for 1 minute. Stop and scrape down the sides of the bowl. On medium low speed, continue to blend for 2-3 minutes more. The batter will be very thick and should look well combined. Pour batter into prepared pans and smooth it out. Bake about 10 minutes (15-20 for full sized cupcakes), checking for doneness with a toothpick. Allow to cool in the pans on a wire rack for 20 minutes.

Now, onto the frosting. In mixer bowl, cream 2-3 tbsp of bacon fat and butter with salt until smooth. Add confectioners' sugar and mix at medium speed until fluffy, about 8 minutes. Add vanilla extract and maple syrup, mixing until you reach desired consistency. Adjust maple syrup and confectioners' sugar to taste.

Frost cupcakes and either roll/dip into the bacon bits or sprinkle them onto the frosting by hand. Drizzle with a little maple syrup if desired and enjoy!

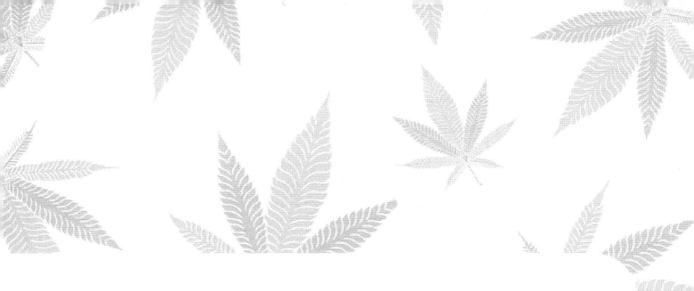

CLOSING QUESTION:

What do I need to know about cooking with cannabis?

Pretty much anything is possible. If it has fat in it, you can medicate it. And, it offers the home cook the advantages of choice, control, customization and cost savings. Cannabutter or oil is the foundation for most recipes (though you can add a bit of activated concentrate instead); it's pretty simple to make and can be substituted or combined in just about any food. Make sure you mix everything well to ensure consistency from bite to bite. And, pay attention to total dosing so you and anyone else enjoying your canna-concoction has a good sense of dosing per serving (and per bite.) Do the math, even if math isn't your thing. You can wing your recipe, but you can't wing dosing.

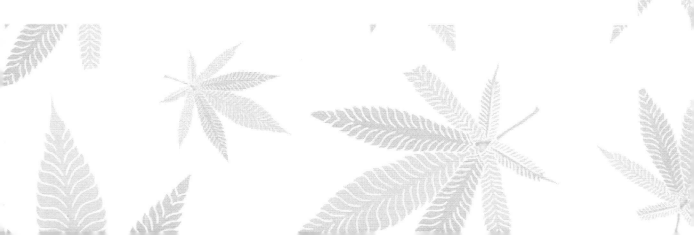

21 | ENTERTAINING AND ENJOYING THE HIGH LIFE

It's the cultural norm to bring a bottle of wine and have a drink when getting together with friends after dark. Adults drink alcohol in social settings to relax, unwind and be more open to new things. Well, cannabis offers the same: it takes the edge off and enhances social experiences.

Now that you're out of the closet, you can start to bring weed into the mix. And not just the Chex mix. From informal get-togethers to fancypants tasting soirees, weed is the guest most everyone loves to have at the table. Mix a group of your best buds with some good food and good bud, and it's a recipe for a good time.

If you're going to invite Mary Jane to the party, here are a few tips to ensure everyone has a good time, but not too good of a time!

BRING POT (IN)TO YOUR NEXT PARTY

How To Be a Good Host

✓ If you're infusing food, use a very light hand when it comes to dosing. Assume more than one or two bites of food will be medicated; you don't want your guests to overdo it. Remember that most recipes assume that's the only medicated food you're eating. Plan ahead and pace the dosing to keep your guests from falling asleep on your couch; you want them to enjoy their night and leave at the end of it!

✓ Have plenty of non-infused food in the mix. You want people to be able to eat well and not worry about getting too high, and to have appealing options for guests who choose not to consume.

✓ Clearly delineate food that is infused and keep it separate from non-medicated food to avoid a mistaken nibble. Make it as dummy-proof as you can. Assume no one will be paying attention to what they're putting in their mouth later in the evening.

✓ If you're offering flower or concentrate for your guests, make sure you have clean gear and all the accoutrements you need...rolling papers, grinder, sanitizing wipes (if you're sharing a vaporizer or bong), a place to empty bowls or place tools. De-stem and de-seed your weed. Always give the first hit to a guest.

✓ Be a responsible host. Educate your guests as needed about going low and slow. Give them a warning about your weed's strength. Tell them to start small. Keep an eye on who's consuming and how they're doing; not everyone knows their limits. Ensure there's a designated driver. Have a plan in place in case someone does overdo it.

✓ Be considerate to your guests and neighbors. If you're going to be smoking joints, try to keep it outside...no one wants to go home smelling like weed. Vaporizing is apartment-friendly and the way to go for anyone concerned with discretion.

✓ Remember that we are all wired differently—one person may have four servings and feel nothing, another guest could have one bite and be off to la-la land. Some will feel it sooner than others; don't let your guests fall into the catch-up trap. Different people will feel different effects; everyone will have their own experience.

✓ And no matter how well you know your guests, do not sneak any medicated food to them. Whether as a prank or a well-intentioned effort to get your mom to try weed, it's not cute, it's not safe and not your choice to make.

✓ If you're lucky enough to be invited as a guest to a pot party, you'll want to be prepared to follow proper stoner etiquette, so that you can get invited back again!

How To Be a Good Guest

✓ Never come empty-handed. If you can, follow stoner tradition and bring some bud of your own to share or as a hostess gift. People who enjoy weed take great pleasure in sharing it with others. You can never go wrong with weed—and you can be pretty sure it won't get re-gifted. If you can't bring weed, bring food. You can't go wrong with that, either.

✓ If joints are being offered, remember it's "puff, puff, pass." Don't slobber and don't bogart the joint. Take your two hits and pass to your left. Keep it moving. And if someone else is bogarting, don't be afraid to break the reverie or monologue and get it moving again.

✓ If there's a bong, the rule of thumb is "hit it and quit it." Clear the chamber before passing to the next person; no one wants your leftover smoke. You don't need to suck down the whole chamber in one hit, nor do you want to and end up with a coughing fit. Take your time and then move it along.

✓ Clean up after yourself—if you're the last one holding the joint, throw it away. If the bowl is cashed, empty it out and repack it. If you knock over the bong (try to avoid this at all costs) clean it up fast. The stink from bongwater sticks around for a long time.

✓ Own your high. Feel comfortable saying "yes" when offered, and feel equally as comfortable saying "no thank you" when you're done. Ask about strength. Know when to say when. Don't be the guest who gets so high you need to take over the guest room. Do be the guest who laughs so hard you snort (or pee…be prepared for bouts of laughter and coughing).

Attend an Elevated Experience: Weed Is the New Wine

Weed is stepping up its game and bringing new appeal to a wider audience through sophisticated events and unique offerings created to bring cannabis to mainstream consumers together in a fun, familiar and safe environment. Marijuana is integrated into the experience, but isn't the primary focus or reason for attending; it's about the overall experience, not showing up to party and get high.

In legal states, you can find high-end events that bring together fine cuisine and cannabis, either as infused dinners or as paired tastings like a wine tasting dinner. There are intimate

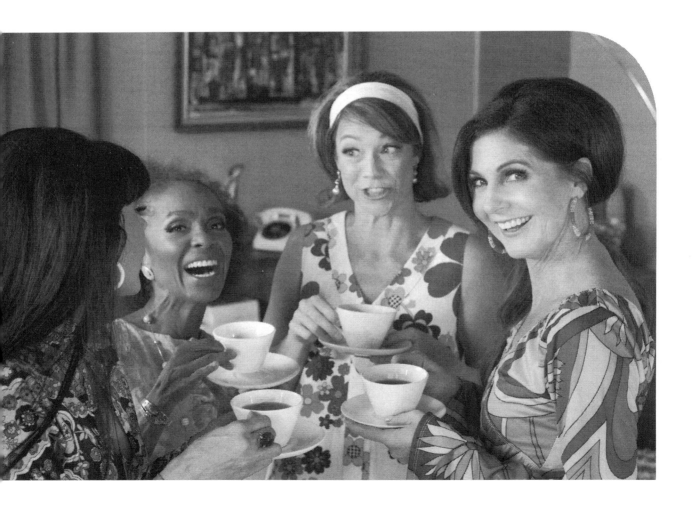

meals prepared by award-winning chefs and tasting parties for growers and brands to show off their finest products. High teas take place in rooftop gardens, and there are mix-and-mingle events for dating, networking and socializing. You generally won't find the old-school stoner stereotypes here.

If you live in or are visiting a state where these events are happening and it works with your schedule or budget, do it. I've been lucky enough to attend a few—when you bring together delicious food, top-notch cannabis and a diverse group of people who share similar interests, your experience is taken to a whole new level. And in states where weed is still underground, there are secret dinner parties and pop-up events—you just have to get lucky enough to score an invitation!

Weed is also making its way into weddings and events, with some setting up cannabis bars with full service budtending, bridal bouquets with buds and bulbs and bud boutonnieres, personalized pre-rolls and other fun party favors to delight and elevate guests. Weed, celebrations and creativity are the perfect combination for a special canna-occasion!

WHEN WEED IS ON THE MENU: TIPS FOR SOCIAL CONSUMPTION

As marijuana makes its way into our lives and into more social occasions, we all have new territory to navigate. People of all experience levels are coming together to celebrate, socialize, connect and perhaps try weed for the first time. So, how do we set ourselves up for the best experience possible?

I asked my good friend, Andrew Mieure of Top Shelf Budtending, best practices for any event in which cannabis is being served. Andrew has been in front of thousands of people at hundreds of events, facilitating their cannabis experience and seeing first-hand what does and doesn't work when it comes to weed and social occasions.

Here are his top tips for inviting Mary Jane to the party:

Respect people's boundaries:
We should be past the point of worrying about peer pressure, but it can still happen even if it's not a group of bros yelling "Chug! Chug! Chug!" There's a fine line between encouragement and peer pressure. Even without external pressure, stepping up to the bud bar can put the pressure on to show how 'cool' we are and lead to overconsumption, which could ruin someone's first (and last) experience with cannabis. Never ever project your enthusiasm or tolerance onto someone else.

Be mindful of set and setting:
Consuming cannabis in your home is very different than in a social setting at a party. Outside of the home is outside of many people's cannabis comfort zone. If you're planning a party, keep this in mind when it comes to your guests. Guest count, venue, aesthetics and comfort all play a huge role in the cannabis consumption experience you're creating. If you're planning to serve joints (a guest favorite) try to designate outdoor space to keep the air as smoke-free as possible...no one wants their clothes to smell like weed after they leave.

Choose cannabis varieties that work well with parties:
Select varieties that dazzle your guest's senses. Choose fruity, citrus and fuel (like diesel) scents for parties that are going to be high energy. If the party is a tad less energetic, provide a few earthy, floral varieties to keep your guests calm and grounded. Always have some low THC (and ideally, high CBD) varieties for guests with low tolerances or who just want to keep it light. There are many more of them than you would think!

Facilitate microservings:
Serve guests intentionally small servings of weed to ensure a smooth experience, particularly if you know many of them are canna-newbs and particularly if you're serving infused food or drink. If you don't know the potency of what you're serving, it's best to be cautious and keep the servings small. Remember, you can always have more, but there are no takebacks once the weed goes into your system. Offering microservings is a sure-fire way to ensure that the guests will have a great time, without getting too high.

Know your guests:
One technique we use at the bud bar is an "experience questionnaire." We ask guests a handful of questions about their cannabis use habits, preferred methods of consumption, allergies and such. This lets us better gauge exactly what each guest requires. Take a little extra time with your guests and with your budtenders, and ensure they give each person their optimal experience. Personalized consumption recommendations for every guest—consuming cannabis at a party will be an absolute delight!

Cleanliness:
For anyone serving or touching cannabis, wear gloves or have a hand-washing protocol in place. Ensure guests have all of the necessary cleaning equipment too, like alcohol pads to wipe down pipes and mouthpieces. Provide ashtrays or other containers for people to cash bowls and dispose of joints. These small cleanliness recommendations aren't only classy, they could prevent sickness. The perception of a clean party alone is worth the price of some gloves and wipes!

The Gauntlet of Going Out in Public

If you're venturing out into the real world while high, gird your loins and prepare yourself inside and out for interacting with the public. I live in a legal state—it's perfectly ok to smell like weed out here. Other places, not so much. For any number of reasons, you might not want to give anyone a hint that you've been hitting a pipe, or whatever form of consumption has gotten you to your happy place. Air yourself out, brush your teeth, Febreeze your space, use some eye drops…whatever you need to freshen up and fly straight.

Be ready to feel like everyone is looking at you and knows exactly what you've been up to. If you're calling attention to yourself and your state of high-ness, it's entirely possible that will actually be true. Case in point: many years ago my friends and I dressed up as Pot Brownies for Halloween while on a girls' weekend in Vegas. We had some cookies that I mistakenly thought were lightly dosed, donned our highly creative costumes and headed out for a nice steak dinner. We were very clearly high and were not being paranoid when we felt all eyes on us. But most of the time, I assure you, it's all in your head. Stay calm and centered, breathe slowly and deeply and repeat to yourself: "It's all in my head; no one is staring at me." (In your head, don't actually say it out loud or you'll turn your paranoia into a self-fulfilling prophecy.)

If You're Going to Mix Weed and Alcohol…

I'm assuming we are all responsible adults, and so let's have an adult conversation about consuming cannabis and alcohol together. First off, there's no physical risk in terms of interactions, unlike many pharmaceuticals. That is not to say that the two together can't make you more wobbly, less clearheaded or otherwise altered if you've gone overboard. Too much of either or both is not a good idea (but too much alcohol is far more dangerous, so make that the thing you keep to a minimum.)

Let's start with what you should know well by now: we are all wired for weed differently. How you respond to the combination will be different than how I do. If you're a canna-newb, don't mix alcohol until you're comfortable with how cannabis affects you. It's important to know what suits your body, and what does not. The wrong combination can turn you into an impaired and unhappy canna-camper, so to speak.

Be aware that the order in which you consume the two could affect how you feel. Weed before alcohol seems to help keep you from getting quite so drunk. On the flip side, alcohol before weed gives your high a turboboost: alcohol significantly increases the THC levels in your blood. If you've had a glass or two of wine, or whatever floats your boat, you're only going to want to take a couple of puffs. Hydrate, hydrate, hydrate. Both weed and booze will dry you out, so drink plenty of water. And since you're a responsible adult, you shouldn't need to be reminded to consume both in moderation!

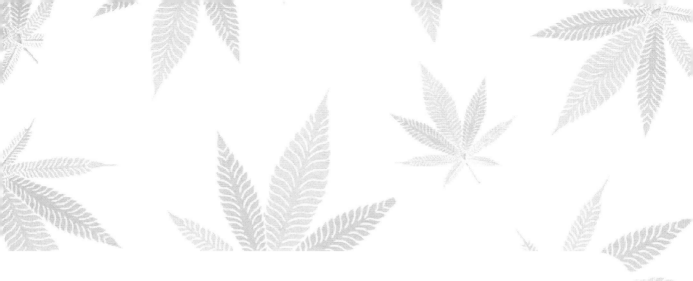

CLOSING QUESTION:

Really... parties, tasting dinners and events with cannabis? How does that work?

Adding weed to a social occasion isn't any different than offering drinks or bringing a bottle of wine. And in reality, weed is a better guest than booze is: cannabis is known to enhance our senses and our palates, not dull them like alcohol can. Weed is being worked into weddings and fancypants events, as well as more 'normal' social occasions like dinner parties and tasting dinners. And why not? It makes experiences better and adds a new way to help people connect and celebrate in new ways!

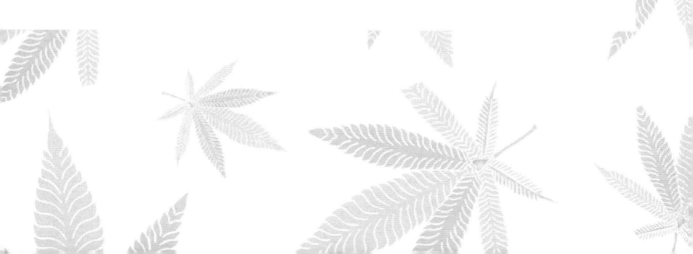

22 | MAKE YOUR NEXT TRIP CANNTASTIC— ELEVATE YOUR TRAVEL EXPERIENCE

Imagine visiting Napa Valley—but with weed instead of wine. Or, imagine Disneyland or Willie Wonka's Chocolate Factory….where anything you can imagine has been "canna-fied" in some way. You can now add weed to the list of things you can try when in Vegas. There are plans to turn a near-ghost town in southeast California into a "cannabis-friendly" resort destination and marijuana-production center. It won't be long until the Emerald Triangle, the Napa Valley of weed, offers the same destination appeal for canna-philes; Humboldt County is practically a brand.

There is an entire industry budding around cannabis tourism in legal states, based on the simple principle we've already covered: everything is better on weed. Cannabis can be integrated into just about any travel plan with delightful results. You can make it a desti-nation getaway with a fully immersive experience, or just add a little extra sparkle to an otherwise normal and non-weed focused trip.

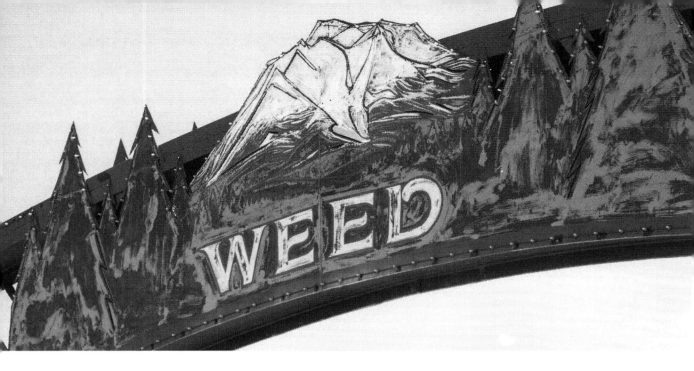

Yes, we now have "pot tour guides" and companies that create customized and packaged experiences that work weed into your weekend plans. The canna-conscious can go to a fully immersive Ganja Yoga retreat with gourmet meals and spa treatments, along with bending and blazing. Before you hit the slopes or head out for a weekend in the mountains, you can hire a weed-friendly charter to help you with whatever provisions you might need.

Chefs will come cook for you (or with you), preparing a delicious multi-course marijuana dinner. Cannabis concierges will help you plan your weekend and then pull all the pieces together for you, so that you don't have to do—or remember—a thing. You can take a foodie tour with pairings and tastings, see a massive marijuana grow operation or take a painting, cooking, sushi-and-joint rolling or glass-blowing class. Or, you can settle into your bud & breakfast, mosey around a cannabis farmers market on a lazy weekend morning, get a cannabis-oil infused massage and just relax and enjoy whatever you're there to enjoy!

But, before you get too excited, even in legal states and more progressive places like Colorado, it's not a free-for-all; there can be a lot of restrictions on where you can consume. Smoking in public can land you a big fine. Most hotels do not allow on-site consumption, even with vaporizers. (Some are more "pot-friendly" than others and take a look-the-other-way approach. Do your research to know where you can consume with confidence and where you cannot.) Respect the local laws and customs, and respect the people around you.

Here are a few dos and don'ts to remember when bringing Mary Jane along on your next trip:

Do

Research before you go

What are the local laws? How much can you buy or carry? What are the rules around public consumption? What do you want to try? Where do you want to shop? What kind of products and strains are available near you? Have an idea of what you want and don't want to help your budtender find what will work best for you. I've given you the foundation, but you need to make it actionable for you.

Have your ID and cash

While you won't be logged into a master marijuana registry, you will need to prove that you are legally able to consume cannabis. If you have a medical card or letter of recommendation, always have that on you. Many dispensaries now take credit or debit cards, but don't count on it unless you've done your homework. Banking is still an issue for many dispensary owners, so it's still largely a cash-based business.

Take your time

Some dispensaries draw crowds and have long lines. Be patient and don't feel rushed or intimidated just because others are waiting. Engage with your budtender. It's your experience. You're allowed to explore your options and ask stupid questions. Or smart questions if you've read the book!

Be honest

Don't be afraid to own up to being a canna-newb. Say it loud and proud: "I have no idea what I'm doing. Please help me." A good budtender will recognize the wonder—or fear—in your eyes and take you through the options best suited for you. You should be getting warnings about your edibles, instructions on how to use the products you're buying and guidance on how best to enjoy whatever you take home with you. Don't just smile and nod. If you don't know what to do or if you have any concerns, speak up!

Plan ahead for where you're going to consume

In all likelihood, you're not going to be able to just walk out the door and spark up a doobie. Smoking a joint is no different than smoking a cigarette, and might just get you fined or booted. Vaporizing is far more discreet, but is still considered public consumption. In some places, people consume quite openly and without hassle (I've been advised to simply "move it along" when an officer passed a group of professional women passing a joint in front of a cannabis business conference). It all depends. Know your options and be prepared so that you're not all weed-ed up with nowhere to go.

Be prepared for the possibilities

If you're new to weed, or are coming to a high-altitude location to get high, be prepared in case you get a little too elevated along the way. Drink lots of water, make sure to keep yourself nourished and hydrated and have some CBD on hand in case you need to bring yourself, or someone you're with, down.

Don't

Buy too much

It's a common mistake tourists make, or even new consumers who suddenly have a wonderland of weed at their fingertips. You can get an ounce for what you pay for a quarter at home! You can't just pick one kind of edible to try! You never have this much choice! Chances are you're going to consume a lot less than you think you will, and unless you're willing to take it home with you (see my answer to the question of whether you can fly with weed), you're going to have a bunch of half-smoked weed or half-eaten edibles on your hands at the end of the trip. Leftover anything is not a tip. I repeat. This is not a tip. Not for your driver, not for the woman who cleans your room. If you leave it, it may be appreciated; don't get me wrong. But it is not equivalent to cash. Make sure you leave some green with any leftover green.

Go overboard

You will want to try everything. It is literally like being a kid in a candy shop. Thousands of products have flooded the market, with more coming every day. Once you decide what type of weed is your thing, you've got to choose how you want to consume it. Gorgeous vaporizers and pipes are available to help you do something with your bud or concentrate. Fancy desktop devices will give you visions of how you can enjoy your herb at home. Anything is possible. Everything is possible. Contain yourself to start, and go back for more once you have your consumption figured out.

Get too high

In wanting to try it all, make sure you don't get too high and take yourself out of the game. Remember the story of my friend who lost two days of her vacation to an edible? It's not just the kids who overdo it and miss the Snoop Dogg concert because they were too high to leave their room. It's not just the edibles that can take you out. A high can creep up on you and suddenly you're stepping into the street without paying attention to the traffic or you feel lightheaded in the middle of a crowd. Take it low and slow and keep your wits about you, especially in a place that's unfamiliar to you. Trust me: there's not much worse than being high and having no idea where you are; it can happen quite suddenly and be very disorienting and scary.

Be indiscreet

Depending on where you are, you can be open and comfortable with consuming cannabis… just don't be too open until you know what's cool and what's not around you. Particularly if you have neighbors, be considerate and sensitive to if kids are around. Know those people who can't handle the excitement of it all? Don't be one of them. Be excited, enjoy (and be) yourself—but be aware of your surroundings and keep it cool, man. Just keep it cool.

Break the law

Or at least if you do so, do it consciously and knowledgeably. Don't be caught by surprise; some places are more lenient than others and others are notoriously strict. Know the local laws and regulations, and in case you get into any trouble, be aware of your rights. Too many marijuana arrests and violations continue to plague our society, make sure you're not one of them.

Get all nervous and worry

Don't stress. The whole point of this is to alleviate stress, right? So if you've made the choice to consume, done your homework to know you can do it with confidence and planned for a good experience, then you've got nothing to worry about. Relax. No one is judging you. No one cares what you're doing. Enjoy yourself, enjoy the company of your people, enjoy the taste of your food and whatever else it is you're doing. Don't worry. Be happy!

Can I Travel With My Weed?

Across state lines, technically no. As long as marijuana remains illegal at a federal level, flying or driving it across state lines, even if both states are legal, is a no-no. This also holds true if you're a medical patient—having a card affords you some protection, but it's not a green light for taking your green anywhere. As I've appropriately disclosed multiple times throughout this book: I do not encourage you to break the law or do something that makes you uncomfortable. What you buy in Vegas, should stay in Vegas. Now, with that said…

The TSA is not looking to bust you for bringing your vape pen or some edibles along on your next trip. The TSA dogs are not trained to search and identify weed. (Customs and Border Patrol dogs are, but unless you're flying internationally, you won't see them sniffing around your bags.) They're looking for bombs, explosives, knives and other dangerous stuff that could kill us. Not the stuff that will chill us out. "TSA security officers do not search for marijuana." Actual words on the TSA website.

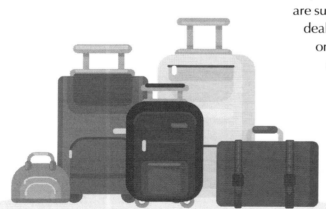

Now, if they do come across it, technically they are supposed to call in local law enforcement to deal with it. But in Denver, where 54 million or so passengers come and go through the airport, there hasn't been a single arrest. And in 2015, only 29 people were even stopped for it during TSA screening. Since the amounts were clearly for personal use, the passengers were simply asked to dispose of it. Everyone complied and that was the end of it. Other local airport authorities handle it differently, so don't assume you'll get off scot-free if you do get caught. But the odds of getting caught are extremely low if you don't make it so obvious that the TSA agent has no choice but to do something about it.

Some patients need to travel with their medicine. Some people simply prefer a little weed instead of a glass of wine or a xanax to take the edge off of flying. For some, it's easier and preferable to travel with their own cannabis, in the form and dosage that works for them. I know quite a few people who frequently travel with weed (in personal amounts of course), and not one has come across a problem yet...even when bags have been opened and checked. Vape pens, edibles and small, securely closed containers of cannabis have all gone through security without issue. This goes for both carry-on and checked bags.

There are endless ways to carry your stash, and thousands of products that are pre-packaged and completely non-obvious once you remove the packaging. Be smart and be cautious, but you have no reason to be paranoid. (But don't get high before screening if you're prone to paranoia. That's just a recipe for disaster.) The bottom line regarding traveling with weed? While it's not without risk, it's not an issue unless you make it one.

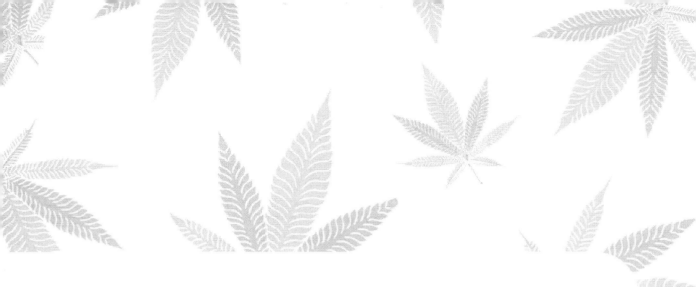

CLOSING QUESTION:

I can take a weed vacation without having to go to Amsterdam?

That's right! (Though if you can get to Amsterdam at some point, by all means, do!) In legal states, pot tourism is turning into big business. From curated, fully immersive experiences to tourist-friendly pot shops, any travel experience can be enhanced with a little weed. Choose from a wide range of activities, classes, tours and experiences, where cannabis can take a starring role or just add a little pixie dust to whatever you're doing. Know what you can and can't do wherever you're going, and act like a responsible adult—you don't want to be the annoying tourist who disrupts everyone else's vacation.

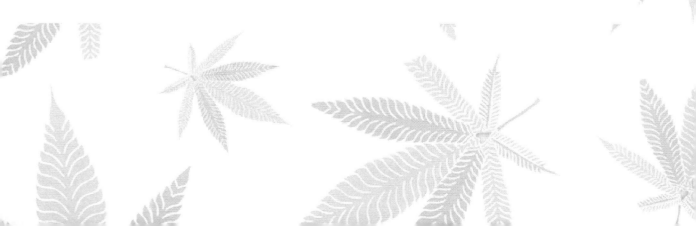

23 | WHEN CANNABIS IS EVERYWHERE: EVERYDAY LIFE, ELEVATED

Once you start to pay attention, you'll see ways weed is—and can be—subtly and seamlessly integrated into everyday life. You'll finally "get it" when you see or hear 420 and get other cultural references and inside jokes. See things from a different perspective. Find ways cannabis could be used in place of meds or alcohol. Seek opportunities to enhance an experience. Meet others who've benefited in some way from bringing cannabis in their lives.

Cannabis is out of the closet. It is becoming the new normal. Stoner Moms are on the Today Show. Retirement communities are forming collectives to grow and create their own cannabis products. Television shows and news programs put the spotlight on weed, entertaining and/or informing us along the way. (Martha Stewart and Snoop Dogg co-host a show—can you believe it?!) Corporate executives are leaving Wall Street for Weed Street. Doctors are forming integrative wellness practices with cannabis as one of many tools available for holistic health and well-being.

Yes, there are still the stoner stereotypes out there in the media and in our culture. Sometimes they're being made fun of; sometimes they're still being embodied. Men have dominated cannabis culture for years, though the landscape is most certainly shifting and women are stepping forward to stake their claim in the spotlight. Media. Entertainment. Fashion. Culture. All of it is undergoing a transformation as weed goes mainstream and the insider culture of cannabis becomes accessible and appropriate for the rest of the world.

It won't be long before mainstream consumers won't put up with the outdated portrayals—not just because it's stale and embarrassingly limited, but because it doesn't represent them. And "them" can mean anyone. Ganja Grannies. Stiletto Stoners. Marijuana Moms. "We" are everywhere, and "we" are nothing like you'd expect.

What does this all mean? That you will start to see yourself, or at least people like you, using weed in normal, everyday ways, where it's not a joke or something requiring stealth and subversion. High society is no longer lowbrow. We already have magazines, TV shows and digital media with cannabis-focused lifestyle and culture content, designed to appeal

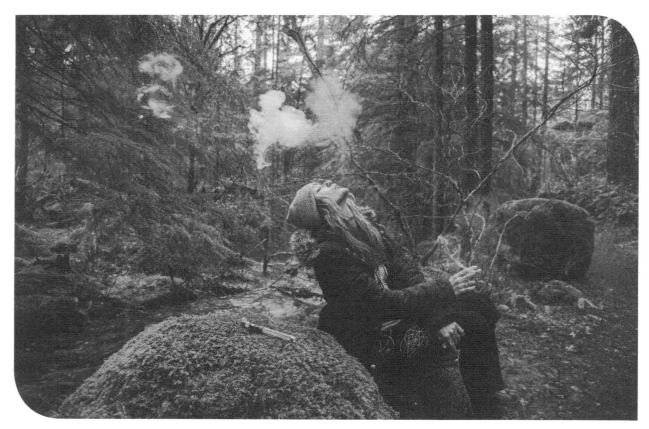

to mainstream and multi-faceted audiences and to elevate the perception of weed and the people who consume it. Advertising is currently very restricted and quite limited, but it won't be long before you start to see ads for cannabis products as you would see for other health, wellness, lifestyle or even alcohol and tobacco brands. There were at least two cannabis companies going after stadium-naming rights in Denver.

And it's not just portrayals and stereotypes; the market is stepping up to meet the new marijuana consumer on her level. Brands and products are being designed both for form and function, targeted to audiences with refined tastes, unique needs and grown-up expectations and budgets. Beyond the design and technology sophistication with vaporizers and other tools for consumption, the world that surrounds and supports the weed consumer is stepping it up, too.

Designer handbags with smell-proof stash spots. Elegant jewelry. Luxury fashion. High fashion offers actual high fashion. Today's cannabista is no longer relegated to outdated hippie fashion. Modern hippie? Yes, of course. But also suburban mom. City hipster and city slicker. Whatever your style, you can find a way to weedify your wardrobe.

LIVE FROM NEW YORK, IT'S CANNABIS COUTURE!

Back in 2016, the exceptionally talented and beautiful actress Margot Robbie opened the season premiere of *Saturday Night Live* in a marijuana leaf Alexander Wang dress. She didn't say a word about weed. It was simply a nod to cannabis and a prime example of the progress our culture is making toward normalization.

Okay, I've Got My Weed. Now What?

If you're looking for ideas on what to do now that you've become all educated about weed and consciously chosen to consume, here are some suggestions and ideas to get the most from getting a little ganja into your life. Even if you're a patient and medicating, there's nothing to say you can't enjoy your experience. Give yourself a pass and take a break from the suffering.

Remember, plan ahead. Make sure you have enough cannabis and all the tools and gear you need to consume it. Have your snacks and provisions on hand, including lots of water. There's nothing more annoying than getting all settled in or ready to go if you're heading out (for some of us, that can take awhile!) and then realizing you forgot something. And then settling back in and realizing you forgot something else. You want to enjoy your experience, not have to keep pulling the pieces together to make it happen.

Choose the strain or product suited for whatever is on tap. Know what works for you and what does not. You don't want to set yourself up for a chill night on the patio with just you and the dog, and get talkative and energetic. No matter how much your dog gets you, he's still not going to engage in a conversation with you. But he'll probably appreciate the extra playtime at least! Or in a reverse scenario, if you're bringing Mary Jane with you to a concert, you don't want to feel like you need a nap in the middle of the show. If you're taking an edible, plan for when the effects are likely to come on and ensure you're not in a situation where you put yourself or others at risk.

Okay, you're ready. You're all set. Let's go!

Make it a TV or movie night

If everything is better on weed, that also means what you're watching is better. Special effects are more spectacular. Silly comedies produce gut-splitting, tear-inducing rides of laugher. Immersive dreamscapes become fully immersive. Visual extravaganzas become extra-awesome. I'm embarrassed to admit I have seen the movie Armageddon more times than I can count while high; it's the only excuse I can offer up, but it is my go-to get-high-and-get-lost flick.

Get lost in the sound

Set up the surround sound or put on your best headphones and immerse yourself in your favorite music. The brain's center for auditory stimulation is triggered by THC, so you can engage more deeply. Turn off the lights, make yourself comfortable and let the sound wash over you. Hear the lyrics in an entirely different way. Some people get so enraptured with the music they feel like they "see" it. Be careful not to get too lost in the sound, though! Back in the day, I was deeply immersed in Pink Floyd's The Wall and was absolutely, positively sure the helicopters were outside my windows. It took me a few minutes to bring myself back to reality and recognize that I was safely and, once I turned down the stereo, quietly ensconced in my room in Ann Arbor. (And yes, I see the irony in this stereotype. It's okay. I embrace that fractal of my whole pot picture!)

Get creative and make something

We've covered weed's ability to inspire and enhance creativity, as demonstrated by so many successful artists. Get inspired and get your hands or head into the act. Have a second childhood and enjoy time for arts & crafts. Paint, draw, take photos, write, brainstorm, or whatever floats your creative boat. Take on a project or pick up a new hobby. I used the focus from my favorite strain, Sour Diesel, to teach myself to knit. My former boss once said she always could tell when I'd written under the influence; and that was a compliment, not a reprimand by the way.

Make a night out of it

Invite friends over for a potluck. Literally. Assign each person a different item to bring (coach them as needed about dosing) or create a theme for the evening. Or host a tasting party, with different strains and pairings for everyone to enjoy. Make it a grown-up only "bake sale" and exchange your favorite edibles. If you aspire to be Martha Stewart, make fancy joints—if origami or paper art of any kind is your thing, you'll be amazed at what can be created with a little spark of inspiration.

Treat yourself (or someone else)

If you've ever enjoyed a glass of wine and a bath, you might really enjoy a little weed with your bathwater. Or rather, before your bath. It's more practical to consume before you get into the tub than to have to deal with wet hands and dropped joints or pipes. Nothing kills a luxurious bath faster than dropping ash into it. If you're lucky enough to have infused bath products on hand (for once, you might actually be happy to have been gifted a bath product!)—what are you waiting for? Drop that dope-soaked thing right in the water and feel your muscles start to melt. If you have infused topicals on hand, get that onto your skin in the most pleasurable way possible. Enjoy how much better everything feels with a little bit of weed!

Get productive

Make your list, gather your tools and supplies and find the strain that makes you get up and go. Get high and then get up and go. You won't even notice that you don't really enjoy doing yardwork or whatever else it is you're doing. You'll find your flow and before you know it, you'll find you're done. And then you can kick back and relax without guilt and with full presence. Everyone wins. How about that?!

Get out there

Don't just stay home: get out there and explore. See your city or town from a different perspective. Stroll around a park or lake and take in the beauty of nature. Go to a museum or gallery. Get lost for a little bit (but make sure it's semi-intentional so you don't suddenly find yourself high and freaking out that you don't know where you are)! Sit outside and gaze at the stars. Whatever you're doing, make sure to chose a strain or product that won't bring out any paranoia once you step outside of the house. No one wants to have a meltdown in the middle of a crowd.

DIY Projects: Get Creative and Express Yourself!

In some cases, there is good reason for a stereotype. We've covered how cannabis is good for creativity and inspiration…you'd be surprised and impressed by the engineering, product design and innovation stoners can apply when properly motivated or inspired.

Whether you broke your glass piece and need to make a homemade pipe (it happens, to some of us quite often!) or want to weed-dazzle whatever your crafty heart desires, you can probably find most of what you need already at home and can most certainly find how-to's, instructions and inspiration online.

Take a peek on Pinterest and get ready to have your mind blown. Bedazzled lighters, handmade jewelry and gifts, needlework patterns. If you can imagine it, you can weedify it. Get a cannabis coloring book and turn it into wall art. Marijuana manicures are even a thing!

And, I promised you earlier I'd show you how to make an apple pipe, so here you go! The next time you're planning to make an apple pie, consider turning one of your apples into a pipe, taking a toke or two and making the prep work fly by.

MAKING AN APPLE PIPE

It's simple and sustainable to boot! Grab an apple, a ballpoint pen/metal straw/something sharp and pokey and get to work:

Remove the stem: Twist off stem of the apple to expose the natural bowl at the top. Get the whole stem out. You're going to be tunneling through that spot.

Make the bowl: Using your poking tool, bore a hole through the top to about midway through the apple. (If using a pen, remove the ink column and cap first.)

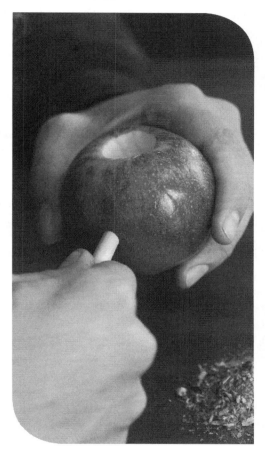

Make the mouthpiece and carb: Pick a spot on the face of the apple as close to the center as possible. Bore another hole completely through the apple, running straight through from one side to the other. The goal is to connect the two chambers; you might need to do a little extra tunneling. You will now have two holes on the side of the apple and one on the top for your bowl.

Load and go: Drop a nug of your favorite bud into the bowl where the stem used to be, put your mouth over one side hole and a finger over the other, and fire it up. It's just like smoking from any other pipe, except that when you're done with this one, you can actually eat it. And no, you won't get high from eating it. An apple pipe doesn't count as an edible.

How To Keep Your Cannabis (and Your Loved Ones) in Good Condition

Proper storage of your cannabis not only keeps it from getting stale and potentially losing its flavor, it keeps it out of the hands (and mouths) of anyone not invited to join you in a sesh. If you have kids or pets at home, it's your responsibility to keep them safe—just as you wouldn't leave pills or booze within reach, the same holds for weed. And if you knock things over like I do, putting everything securely away when not in use will also keep it from being lost to spillage or breakage.

If you're keeping flower at home, don't keep it in a plastic bag. It's fine for transport or short-term storage, but you want to store flower in airtight containers. Mason jars and glass screw-top jars, or jars specifically made for storing cannabis, work best. Ideally you want as little extra air space in there as possible; too much air leads to excessive dryness. And we can all appreciate wanting to avoid excessive dryness!

Perhaps you'll want an elegant coffee table showpiece that holds your cannabis and the tools you need to enjoy it. Or maybe it's a lockable bag that carries the gear you want to take on the go or tuck out of sight. Whatever fits your lifestyle and your home situation, there's something out there for every cannabis user to carefully and securely keep their stash. You're a grown-up. No more baggies and bits of weed everywhere. Got it?

Know Your Rights

Remember, cannabis is still illegal in the United States. Despite the number of states that have legalized it in some form (and even more that have decriminalized possession), it's possible you could get into trouble for your cannabis. It could be a misdemeanor or felony, depending on amounts and other factors such as where you were caught and what you were doing (and sadly, in some places, the color of your skin). Penalties can run from license suspension and fines to jail time.

If you have a medical card, carry it on you always. It's by no means a get-out-of-jail-free card, but it does afford you some protection. If you're traveling, check reciprocity laws. Generally speaking, if you're a responsible adult who doesn't make your consumption a public nuisance, you'll avoid trouble.

But there are exceptions and if you do have an encounter with the law, admit nothing. Stay quiet. Never consent to a search. Without a warrant or probable cause (which means drugs or paraphernalia in plain sight), you are not obligated to consent. Refusing a search is not an admission of guilt and does not give an officer a right to search you. And if you're not being detained, you are free to go. If you are formally detained, repeat step one and get a lawyer. Admit nothing. Stay quiet and stay calm. Do not chat it up.

Oh, and when it comes to employers and weed; their rules go. You can get fired for failing a drug test, even if you are in a legal state and even if you have a physician's recommendation. If you are concerned about drug testing, there's no magic formula to knowing how long THC will stick around your system. It depends on metabolism and how much THC is hanging around—the more you consume, the longer it will be detectable. The general guideline is that one-time usage is detectable in blood for 12-24 hours and in urine for one to seven days. Regular users show evidence for two to seven days in blood and from one week to three months in urine. As to whether you can cheat a drug test? All I will say is that many people do. As to how? All I will say is to use the Google and proceed at your own risk. (And use good judgment; do your homework!)

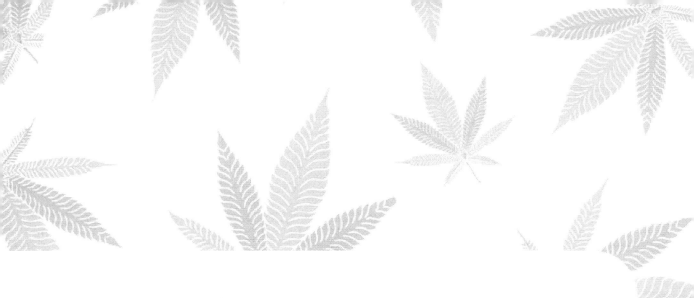

CLOSING QUESTION:

What do I do with myself once I actually consume my cannabis?

Weed can be worked into everyday life with ease, once you figure out what works for you. It is already being integrated into our culture and society, it's just not that big of a deal anymore. You can use cannabis to enhance experiences, de-stress, disconnect with the mayhem of life and connect with what and who is important to you, get playful and silly or simply to have fun. Used mindfully and responsibly, however you use cannabis, for whatever reasons, it's all good!

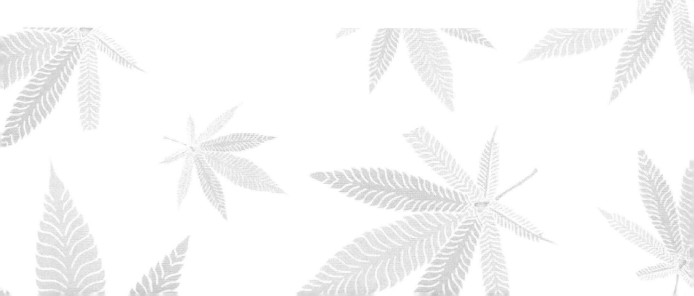

24 | HOME GROWING AND MAKING YOUR MEDICINE

In my 20s, I thought growing your own marijuana was as simple as throwing a seed from my bag of weed into a cup and letting my garden grow. Yeah, that's not how it works. I got my seed to grow into a sprig with a leaf identifiable enough to spark the conversation with my mom; but it never developed buds or turned into anything usable. (Apparently to flower, marijuana plants need light in cycles of 18 hours. Who knew?!) At one point, I plucked the leaves and tried to get high. It didn't work.

Gardening is not my thing, and so unlike just about every other aspect of weed, I have no first-hand experience with growing marijuana. I am good friends with unbelievably skilled growers, I let them do all the work and get straight to the output of their efforts. But there are plenty of experts and resources out there, so if you're looking to go deeper than a basic overview of growing marijuana, you won't have to figure it out on your own. Lots of people before you have figured it out and are happy to share their expertise and opinions!

If you love to garden, growing your own cannabis can be therapy in and of itself. Tending to your "girls," as the plants are called, takes a lot of TLC. Even if THC isn't your thing, you can grow high-CBD strains and still reap all the benefits without the high. But, if you are going to grow cannabis at home, you've got to do more than throw a seed into a cup and water it now and then.

There are many ways to bring a marijuana plant from a seed to your shelf, so you've got to go through some thought and planning before you can get to growing. Where and how will you grow? Indoors or outside? Do you have a safe and secure place to grow? What light will you use? What do you need to consider in terms of legality, neighbors and available space/resources? What supplies and equipment will you need to buy? How committed are you to nurturing and tending to your plant(s)? Growing your own cannabis takes time and investment, no matter which way you go with your grow.

Here are three key questions you'll want to answer before getting started:

1 What strain(s) do you want to grow?

What are you looking to treat and/or what effects are you seeking from your cannabis? Start with the desired end result and select the strain(s) most likely to deliver. Different strains mature at different rates; if you're growing more than one strain, you'll need to manage their growth cycles. Indicas and indica-dominant hybrids are generally easier for beginners to grow, have shorter flowering cycles and higher yields. Indicas take eight to 12 weeks in flowering stage; sativas can take 12 to 14 weeks.

2 Are you starting from seed or clone?

You can buy clones from many dispensaries, or take cuttings from another plant and grow your own with identical characteristics of its mother. If you're taking a cutting from someone else's plant, make sure it's in the vegetative or "veg" state and not developing any buds yet.

You can also start from seeds. And yes, you can also buy seeds online, if you can believe it! As long as they come from outside the U.S. (and from a reputable seed bank), it's safe and reliable. Seed banks also come with the added advantage of letting you know what to expect, how long to wait before harvest, whether the strain is suited for indoor or outdoor growing and what effects to expect from the finished product. Unless you want to be dealing with monitoring your garden for male (or hermaphrodite) plants, which must be removed immediately, make sure you get sinsemilla (seed-free female) plants.

3 Are you growing indoors or outside?

This is probably the most important question to answer, as it drives every aspect of your grow and possibly your timing. If you have access to plenty of sunlight, even if it's on a balcony or patio, you can grow outdoors. Plan for May through November as your growing season. It's less expensive and less work, and more environmentally sound. And natural sunlight is hard to beat—plants tend to grow bigger outside. Of course, sunlight doesn't negate discretion or provide protection, so factor in nosy neighbors, pesky critters and other considerations if you're thinking about sungrown cannabis. You only get one shot during growing season, so it's do or die until next year.

If you take it inside and grow indoors (or "indo" in shorthand), you'll need to create a designated space and bring in lighting and other materials to support your grow. You will need a spot that can be completely dark for 12 hours for extended periods of time. If you don't have a dedicated space to turn into a grow room, you can buy a portable grow tent or other device designed specifically for an out-of-the-box home-grow solution.

Depending on how serious you get, you may need to upgrade your electrical supply; or add cooling and ventilation systems to keep the conditions inside right, and the nosy neighbors on the outside *all right*. With indoor grows, you control the conditions and are less exposed; plus you have the advantage of growing when it works for you or year-round harvests, take your pick! But they're also more expensive (lights, electricity, AC and equipment all cost money) and take more work.

—

Regardless of which way you go, make sure you can keep your grow safe and secure from kids, nosy neighbors or potential ne'er-do-wells who could put you and your grow at risk.

10 Easy Steps to Get Growing

Once you've figured out your approach and what you'll need to get going, it's time to get growing! You will nurture your plant(s) for four months through distinct phases of growth, giving her light and nutrients so she'll flourish and produce big, sticky buds. Here are the fundamental steps to get you started—once you master the basics, you can start to experiment with more sophisticated grow techniques and equipment such as lighting if you want to get serious about home cultivation.

1 Select your strain
What are you looking to treat and/or what effects are you seeking from your cannabis? Start with the desired end result and select the strain(s) most likely to deliver. If you're lucky enough to know another grower or have access to clones or seeds through a dispensary or collective, you can generally trust the quality of what you are receiving. Whether you go with an indica strain, a sativa strain or a hybrid strain, be sure you get feminized seeds—it's only the female plants that have all the magic going on. Let's hear it for the ladies!

2 Pick your pot
Start with a container about the same size as a five-gallon bucket and be sure it has plenty of drainage holes. You want plenty of oxygen to reach the roots as your little girl grows up. Go with either a deep gardening pot, a fabric pot or a sturdy bucket with holes drilled into the bottom. The key thing here is that you don't want your plant sitting in a bunch of soggy, undrained soil—this could damage her roots or lead to mold.

3 Settle on your soil
The easiest growing medium for beginning cannabis growers is a good, organic potting-soil mix. These soils usually contain a mix of nutrients and other stuff designed to keep the soil light and airy. Look for things like coco fiber, compost, earthworm castings, bat guano, peat moss, and kelp meal. Stay away from anything with "extended" or "slow release" nutrients. Don't pack the soil down—you want it to stay fluffy so your roots don't have any trouble getting nutrients or growing.

4 Sprout that seed

Gently plant the seed ½ to 1 inch deep. Cover it with a light layer of soil and lightly water it until the soil is thoroughly moist. Put it in a warm place and keep it moist until you see your baby sprout—don't let the soil dry out, but don't overwater and drown your seed. The first leaves will be rounded and won't look like marijuana leaves. You didn't get the wrong seed or do anything wrong. Give it some time. Soon you'll see the first, tiny recognizable marijuana leaves.

5 Let there be light

Once you see baby leaves appear, it's time to move your plant into the vegetation stage (called "veg" by the pros) by giving it light. Lots of light. Light management is critical at this stage in your girl's development. Whether through sunlight or indoor lighting, you want her getting 18 hours of light a day. (If you're going to become a serious grower, you will want to research and invest in professional indoor lighting at some point.) This is time when your plant is putting all her energy into putting down roots and growing into a big, bushy, strong and healthy plant.

6 Sit tight and feed her right

Your plant won't bud for a few more months, so now is the time to just keep giving her lots of light and high-quality organic fertilizer. This is the longest and most important phase of your plant's life. Be patient and give her plenty of TLC as she grows up. Use plant food throughout the growing phase to give your young plant the nutrients she needs. Ideally, get some plant food that's been specially formulated for the specific needs of cannabis plants. As she begins to grow, be sure you keep her well watered, but not too wet. After watering, wait until the top inch of soil dries out before watering it again. Don't over-water and don't go overboard with the nutrients. Keep her comfortable, 70–85° F (20–30°C) is ideal.

Keep an eye out for mold, spots, disease, pests or fungus and carefully remove any damaged leaves. Keep your hands off the plant as much as possible, and be gentle when you do handle her; she's sturdy but still can be damaged. When your plant has reached the desired size, it's time to start her flower cycle.

7 Fire up the flowering

Outdoors, the long days of summer start to give way to the shorter days of fall, which triggers the flowering phase. Indoors, you'll start to reduce the light and give her a longer "night." Her day will consist of 12 hours of light and 12 hours of darkness. Soon, you'll start to see her buds appear. It's just a little longer now!

8 Ready, set, harvest!

As your plant begins to flower, you'll see the buds start to show their trichomes: those sticky, hair-like things with tiny crystals on the tips...that's where all the good stuff is. They start off clear and when nearing readiness to harvest, they turn milky-white and translucent. You're almost there. When they turn amber, that's the magic moment. Be patient. You want to wait until she's really ready to be harvested. The longer you wait, the higher the quality and smoother and more potent the finished product will be. Carefully cut the buds off at the stem, making sure you don't damage the actual buds. Remove any large stems or leaves (this all becomes trim, which you can use in further extraction and processing).

WHY IS THERE A "NO BOYS" SIGN POSTED?

No hate, but you only want girls in your garden. It's the unpollinated female cannabis plant that delivers all the cannabinoid goodness we've been talking about; instead of producing seeds, she puts all her energy into trichome production. If you find any males hiding during the early flowering stage, you must kill them before they begin to mature and spread their seeds. It's not cold-blooded, it's just how it has to be!

9 Hang it high to dry

Fresh bud is a fantastic thing to behold, but it won't do you any good until you dry it enough to cure properly so that you can bring all your hard work over the finish line. To dry freshly harvested bud, tie strings to the stems and hang them upside down in a well-ventilated room. Check a few times a day to see how dry the buds are getting. When the smaller stems get dry enough to easily snap in half, it's time to move onto the curing phase.

10 Cure until it's consumable

Curing your weed is the key to getting the best flavor and the most potency from your plant. Don't underestimate how strong the aroma is, be prepared for that infamous skunk smell to permeate the space. The simplest way to do it? Remove the buds from the larger stems, place all those dried buds into glass mason jars and screw on the lids. You don't want them crammed in, but you don't want a lot of air in there either. Keep the jars in a dark place, and check their moisture content once or twice a day. Too moist? Let it air out a bit. Keep checking until the buds are nice and perfectly sticky without being too sticky-icky. Once you've got that perfect balance, your bud is ready for whatever you have planned for it!

—

Sit back and enjoy the fruits of your labor! And be sure to take a moment to give gratitude to the plant and what she will bring to your life—you two worked hard together to produce this harvest.

If You Want to Make Your Medicine...

For many people, and medical patients in particular, it may be more effective and, in large quantities, far less expensive to make your own tincture or cannabis oil. It gives far greater control and customization over the end product: from the strain profile and cannabinoid ratios to potency and dosing. And, it's probably far easier than you think.

Cannabis Tinctures

Let's start with tinctures. Cannabis tinctures were legally sold as medicine in the U.S. until 1937, until along came Reefer Madness. Marijuana-infused ethyl alcohol, usually dispensed via an eyedropper, is easy to titrate, low in calories and boasts a long shelf life—many years when stored in a cool, dark location. Although edibles are the most popular way to consume marijuana without actually smoking it, they can be hard to dose and have to be consumed relatively quickly. Tinctures offer give you the convenience of a long shelf life and control over dosing, and give you the flexibility to directly drop into your mouth or add to food or drink.

Making cannabis tincture at home is simple and relatively mess- and fuss-free. All you really need is a jar, high-proof alcohol, a strainer and, of course, weed! You'll also want a funnel and medicine dropper bottle(s) for the final product.

1 First you have to grind and decarboxylate your weed. Grind finely and bake at 225 degrees in an oven-safe tray for 30–45 minutes. Let it cool for about 30 minutes.

2 Grab your mason jar and fill it with high-proof alcohol. Everclear or Bacardi 151 is a good choice. Mix in your weed, close the jar and shake it up. Vigorously.

3 Now, depending on your philosophy and/or patience, you will let the jar sit anywhere from a few minutes to a few months. You can shake the mixture for three minutes and move on to strain and store it. Or, you can put it on a shelf in a cool, dark place and shake it once or twice a day for up to three months. (Apparently you can also give the mixture a little water bath in its jar for 20 minutes at 170 degrees and shortcut the whole three-month shake weight workout.)

4 Strain the mixture through a cheesecloth or coffee filter, squeezing as much as you can through to get all those juicy cannabinoids. Transfer to a medicine dropper bottle(s) to protect the tincture from light; store in a cool, dark place for a long shelf life.

Start with 1mL of your finished tincture and put it under your tongue. If you're happy with the effects, you're done. Otherwise, try 2mL the next day and so on until you find the volume you're happy with (ramp up slowly while testing your desired dosage so you can avoid getting uncomfortably high).

Cannabis Oil

Medical cannabis oil is made from the buds and sometimes leaves of the cannabis plant and can be highly therapeutic. You might know it as Rick Simpson Oil (RSO), Phoenix Tears or hash oil. This is not the same as CBD oil, which is made from industrial hemp and does not contain the same array of beneficial cannabinoids and terpenes. A ful-extract cannabis oil contains a diverse amount of cannabinoids and maintains the integrity of the whole plant.

Rick Simpson Oil has become quite famous in the past decade because of widespread claims it can cure cancer and a wider spectrum of mental as well as physical ailments. Many patients claim to have found success in treating cancer, epilepsy, multiple sclerosis and numerous other difficult-to-treat medical conditions. I'm not here to substantiate or debunk these claims; as I've said, I'm not a doctor, and there's no source out there that will validate or verify what people believe or have experienced. I'm not making these claims; though many others are. And I'm certainly not claiming or promising that it will heal or treat whatever ails you or a loved one. That said, some people have found it to be beneficial and so, as I advise with everything else, use common sense in considering whether cannabis oil is a path for healing.

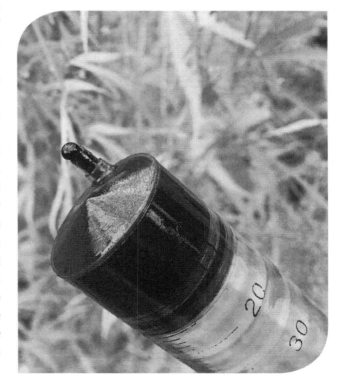

Beyond cost savings, the key advantage of making your own cannabis oil is the ability to control the strain and cannabinoid profile of your extract: what goes in comes out in highly concentrated form with the same characteristics. Each individual and medical condition responds best to different types of cannabis. For example, strains high in both THC and CBD are thought to work well in cancer treatment. Seizure disorders, however, respond better to high-CBD, low-THC strains. High-THC plants could produce levels in excess of 60%, resulting in a very psychoactive effect. High-CBD plants deliver extracts with no high. More and more people favor strains with a 1:1 ratio of THC to CBD, as research suggests the two work best when combined with each other, and not separated. Remember that CBD tames THC's psychoactivity, so if it's in the extract, any psychoactivity will be minimal.

Making cannabis oil at home is relatively easy, using grain alcohol as the solvent for extraction. That said, it does involve heat and flammable liquids, so be prepared and have a fire extinguisher on hand. Make sure you're working in space that's well ventilated, ideally outside.

You'll need:

  – One ounce of high-quality cannabis (or two to three ounces of trim)

  – Everclear alcohol

  – Double boiler

  – Medium glass mixing bowl

  – Cheesecloth or clean nylon stocking

  – Large wooden spoon

  – Silicone spatula

  – 2-quart mixing cup or container (to catch liquid)

  – Sterile oral syringes

  – Cooking thermometer

  – Fans or ventilation (if indoors)

  – Parchment paper

1 Perform solvent extraction

Using high-proof alcohol as a solvent eliminates any potential carcinogens. The alcohol completely burns off in the cooking process, leaving you with nothing but pure, extremely concentrated cannabis oil. Here's how you extract with your solvent:

- Add your cannabis to your glass bowl.

- Pour your alcohol into the bowl, just enough to cover the herb.

- Stir the cannabis with your wooden spoon continuously for a couple of minutes.

2 Strain and soak

Strain out the plant material from the solvent. (You're going to repeat the extraction process a second time).

- Cover your 2-quart measuring cup or extra container with cheesecloth or a clean nylon stocking (make sure you can easily grab and bundle up your strained material.)

- Pour the cannabis mixture over the cheesecloth into the second container.

- Gather up the cheesecloth or nylon and squeeze out the remaining liquid.

The dark-green liquid is now a mixture of alcohol and extracted cannabis resin. The first soak removes the majority of the cannabinoids, the second soak gets the rest.

- Take your strained plant material and empty it back into your glass mixing bowl.

- Pour more Everclear over the top until it is fully submerged.

- Stir continuously with your wooden spoon for a couple of minutes.

- Repeat the straining process and empty your second batch of alcohol into your runoff container.

3 Heat and separate

Now it's time to separate the cannabis resin from the solvent with heat. Remember, safety is key here. Make sure that you have as much air circulation and ventilation as possible to avoid any mishaps. You want all of the fumes to head outside. Ideally you want to be outside. If you're indoors, keep your air moving. The last thing you want is an explosion in your kitchen.

- Fill the bottom of your double boiler with water.

- Pour canna-alcohol into the top pan.

- Turn your burner on high and wait for your top pot to boil.

- Once the liquid bubbles, immediately turn off your burner. The boiling water will do the rest.

- Let the mixture in the top pan bubble for 15 to 20 minutes. You can turn the burner back on if you stop getting bubbles.

- Once the oil is nice and thick, it is complete. Remove it from the pan and scrape it out onto parchment paper when it cools.

4 Fill syringes

When the oil has cooled, you can suck up your cannabis oil into your syringe for proper dosing. You can also use a syringe to fill new, empty pill capsules to make your own cannabis pills.

People use this oil directly on their skin or ingest it in various amounts. The oil can be eaten on a piece of toast with your favorite spread (or anything that can mask the taste) or can be put into an empty capsule. If you don't mind the taste, you can place it under your tongue for the most efficient absorption. Don't forget about suppositories as well—for patients with cancer in their digestive system, this is the most effective path for absorption. You can get cocoa butter and a mold and make suppositories with the oil as a fifth step. Generally speaking, getting the medicine as close to the source of the problem as possible is best.

Rick Simpson developed a course of treatment that many cancer patients follow in an effort to eradicate the disease—60 grams of cannabis oil ingested over roughly 90 days. The program starts with small doses and builds up to 1 gram/day.

The treatment starts with three doses of oil per day. For the first week each dose is the size of a half grain of white rice. After a week, double the dose. Continue doubling every four days until 1 gram (or 1 ml) per day is ingested. Most people to get to the point where they can ingest 1 gram per day in 30–35 days. Once 1 gram of oil per day is achieved, dosage continues at that level for another 60 days or so. Some people have daily doses to 2 grams or more. Some stay on the treatment longer. Everyone responds differently.

Dosing the oil slowly over the first 30 days allows the body to build up a tolerance. If using a CBD-rich oil, the lack of psychoactivity may speed the ability to increase dosing and get to the 1 gram/day target. People who do experience a "high" or extreme tiredness during the day can slightly reduce the dosage during daytime hours and slightly increase the dosage before bed.

Once the course of treatment ends, it's recommended to continue with dosing of 1 gram per month to maintain health and well-being.

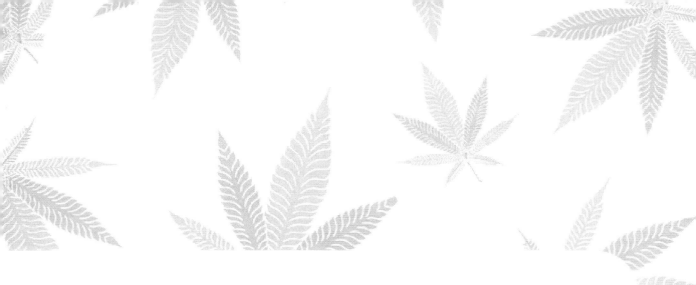

CLOSING QUESTION:

What are the advantages of growing or making my medicine?

When you grow or make concentrated cannabis oil at home, you get a lot more control over what you're consuming. Perhaps most importantly, you get to choose the strain that will deliver the effects and cannabinoids you want. And, once you get done with the set-up costs, it's far more cost effective for anyone who consumes in quantity. Patients who use cannabis oil will certainly find this less expensive than paying per-gram pricing on the market, though collectives and other patient-centric organizations may have affordable options. For those with a green thumb, it can be a fun new hobby, for those in need of serious medicine, if you have the space, this may be a good option to consider.

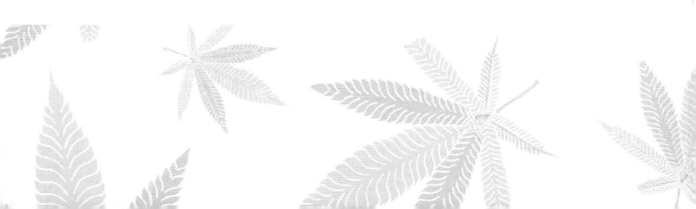

25 | ON CANNABIS & COMMON SENSE: CLOSING THOUGHTS AND PARTING WISDOM

Before I wrap it up and let you get going, first I'd like to take a moment to thank you. Thank you for being open-minded and interested in something you've probably been led to believe is bad—very, very bad—for the vast majority of your life. Thank you for taking time to educate yourself and form your own opinions. I have mine; I don't make any bones about my subjectivity. Thank you for listening to what I have to say. Even if you don't agree with all or any of my points, you're here. You're willing to consider a conversation, even if it's only with yourself at this time.

I've given you a lot to digest. We may have years of deep-rooted perceptions and stigma still to work through and unravel. It's okay, I don't expect you to just embrace weed in all its glory and potential and join the "cult of cannabis." Take it all in, and take it slowly. Dip a toe in the water. Start to be more aware of opportunities where cannabis could provide relief. Replace a pill or a drink. Enhance an experience. Or dive in—whatever floats your boat! No matter what you want to get from weed, anything is possible.

Weed isn't for everyone, but I do think everyone should approach it with an open mind and that more people should give it a chance. It is not a miracle drug that can cure everything and everyone—but for many people, it produces miraculous results. I cannot count how many times I've heard someone say: "I just didn't notice my pain anymore; it's a miracle!" The word can be used in many ways, and depending on your situation, it might just actually turn out to be true.

As I've emphasized throughout the book, I'm not a doctor, nor do I play one on TV. I'm not giving you medical advice or promising you results. If you're considering medical marijuana to treat a condition, talk to your doctor. Ideally, talk to a doctor trained and focused on medical cannabis and integrative wellness. Even if you don't live in a legal state, many doctors will schedule a remote consult to help answer your questions and go deeper into your therapeutic and medical needs. The vast majority of our medical professionals have not been brought up to speed or trained in medical marijuana and how to integrate it with traditional medicine. Many are still closed off to the concept of marijuana as medicine; others are open but have no knowledge or direction for actually using it. You have the power in your hands to heal, but you have to take control over your health. You have to be an active participant. You have to arm yourself with the knowledge and information you need to make the right decisions for you and your loved ones. As overwhelming at it can be, when it comes to your health, it really is all on you.

If you or your doctor wants solid proof and comprehensive backup, we're just not there yet. Credible information is starting to come forward, but it will be years before modern science can back up ancient wisdom and (substantive) anecdotal evidence. I didn't make up (or back up, for that matter) the data or proof points I use to make my case; all of it is out there on the google. I'm not presenting my case to a peer-review journal or medical board. I researched and synthesized vast amounts of information, filtering it through my lens to make my case to you (or perhaps your family) as to why cannabis should be looked at with fresh eyes and an open mind.

My mom always wanted me to be a lawyer; clearly I chose another path. But, I've been told I can make a pretty good case, even if it's not in a court of law. So, allow me to take this opportunity to recap my common-sense case for cannabis to you and anyone else who might be waking up to weed and its many possibilities:

The fundamental principle that marijuana is a gateway to raging addiction and bad behavior, that it's dangerous and bad, is simply wrong.

Really. Go back and read the first section. We have objective evidence. The only reason we think weed is bad is because we've been programmed to fear it by white men with political agendas and personal biases, who vilified marijuana and the people who consume it. They both completely disregarded objective, scientifically-backed commissions that not only found marijuana is not bad, but also recommended it should be legalized. And today, we have a system that hasn't caught up with modern thinking or science. Cannabis has been used as medicine and as part of our culture for thousands of years, for thousands of reasons. Step back and look at it from a higher perspective.

It cannot be denied that for some people, marijuana provides real and sometimes life-changing benefits.

There is enough evidence to know that there is *some* medical value in marijuana. Kids don't just stop having seizures. Patients do find legitimate relief from marijuana, even if we're not sure yet about the healing part. People dependent on opioids do use marijuana as an exit drug. Sufferers of PTSD do find some peace. Credible doctors and scientists confirm it does have promise. Our bodies are wired for weed. Literally. Like a lock and key. This isn't just coincidence. It means something.

Unlike prescription drugs and alcohol, weed isn't addictive or deadly.

You cannot overdose. Not one person has died from too much pot. Our country is racked with an opioid epidemic; even the president was forced to acknowledge it. (Of course, the government continues to deny the increasingly well-known ability for weed to actually get people off pills, and so that acknowledgment offers little real hope for those who suffer from addiction.) Weed can take on the top five prescription drugs, offering a natural alternative without the side effects and interactions. Any side effects from marijuana are limited, and are generally manageable and preventable. And weed is safe—far, far safer than pills or booze.

The fact that marijuana remains a Schedule 1 substance defies any rational thinking.

We have the FDA asking for public input on CBD, a government patent on CBD for its therapeutic potential and 29 states (plus Washington DC) that support the medical value of marijuana for patients with certain conditions. Let's go over the definition of a Schedule 1 drug again: 1) it has no potential for abuse; 2) it has no currently accepted medical use in treatment in the U.S.; and 3) there is no accepted safety for use, even under medical supervision. No, no and no! Flat-out false on all fronts. Just let the hypocrisy wash over you for a minute.

On the subject of abuse, addiction and dependency, I will say while marijuana is not physically addictive, it can be abused in the same ways other substances are used as crutches or tools to manage pain and trauma.

If you or someone you love is inclined to this kind of behavior, weed isn't going to fix an unhealthy relationship with yourself or others; but it might just help break a life-threatening physical addiction. If depression is a factor, choosing the right product and staying intentional with consumption can keep the therapeutic potential of cannabis on the table and ensure weed isn't contributing to the situation. When all is said and done, weed isn't the problem—but the relationship some people have with it can be. Proceed with caution if this is an area of concern.

Used mindfully, consciously and responsibly, weed can play a beneficial role in many people's lives.

Medically, therapeutically and even recreationally—'better' is simply better, however it's defined. Pain. Sensory experiences. Seizures. A host of medical conditions. Sex. Food. There's truth to the claim that "everything's better on weed." There is nothing wrong with wanting to feel good and add a little sparkle to an experience. It's okay to get silly. I remember my uber conservative ex at his happiest when I finally got him to break down his barriers and smoke a few bowls with me while on vacation. Let loose now and then. Go ahead and give it a whirl.

If you're freaked out about getting too high, or about getting high at all, relax.

You have plenty of options to get the benefits you do want from cannabis, without the psychoactivity you don't want. And if you're paranoid about paranoia and anxiety, remember that you have plenty of options to mitigate that risk. Weed may be stronger than it was in our youth, but there are also plenty of low-THC and high-CBD strains and products for the cannabis consumer who's not looking for max thrust in their experience. It's a whole new world of weed out there, people. You can now literally take a chill pill.

If you're freaked out about your neighbors, friends or family knowing that you've chosen to consume, you have plenty of choices that allow discretion.

Vape pens, edibles, tinctures and even patches no one can see. But before you confine yourself to the cannabis closet, ask if it's really necessary. The stigma may be sticky but the majority of people support legalization and safe access. Cannabis is becoming accepted in our communities and our lives.

Don't be afraid to come out of the closet, own your decision and be confident in your choice. But if your choice is to keep it on the down low, you've got plenty of options. They'll never know…

Weed is not one-size-fits-all.

We are all snowflakes and cannabis is an incredibly complex plant with hundreds of cannabinoids and countless combinations of therapies and effects. It may kill tumors in one person and make another violently ill. It can be used as a numbing tool that keeps you in the energetic muck, or it can be the key to taming your anxiety or sending a bolt of inspiration that gets you moving forward. Some will use it to break addictions, others as medicine. Some will use it mindfully, to connect with their bodies, minds, hearts, spirit and loved ones. Others will use it therapeutically to disconnect with trauma, anxiety and depression. Everyone will get value from cannabis for different reasons. In different ways. With different effects. When it comes to weed, it truly is all about you.

Don't let fear keep you from moving forward.

I hope I've knocked out the misperceptions and misinformation to set the record straight on the facts vs. myths. You can't overdose or die from weed. You won't become a drug-fueled maniac, finding yourself at orgies and behaving in ways you or your family would find shocking. You won't turn into the stereotype. If you've had a bad experience, you shouldn't assume it will happen again. There are products and techniques to mitigate all the stuff you don't want. I've given you all the information you need to choose wisely and keep yourself in check (repeat after me: low and slow, low and slow.) Far fewer people are judging the people who do consume. The authorities generally don't care about your weed, unless there's something else going on. Just toke up and chill out, dude.

Cannabis is not a drug; it's a plant. It's natural, safe and has been around for thousands of years. It is the great equalizer, bringing people of different ages, races, backgrounds and perspectives together, creating a shared experience and connection that bridges perceived barriers and boundaries. Cannabis can help heal. Not just people (and pets). Communities. Relationships. Our planet. Weed can, in many ways, make the world a better place.

You may not share my passion for the potential and power of this plant, but you do have to appreciate her versatility and variability. A single plant can replace multiple pharmaceutical drugs (Big Pharma most definitely doesn't share my passion on this point!). Wean people from addiction and dependency and replace harmful substances like alcohol and tobacco (more big business threatened by this one little plant). It can enhance experiences and bring joy and pleasure. (Again, I ask: what is wrong with that?)

All I ask is that you separate judgment from ingrained perception; real information from propaganda. Please, dig deeper into whatever piece of information you're questioning or concern you may have. This is a general "field guide" to weed—I'm giving you a lot of information (filtered through my lens, to be clear), but what you do with it is on you.

If I've made my case effectively and knocked out most of the barriers, what's left is the question of whether cannabis is right for you or a loved one. What role, if any, could weed play in your life? I can't answer the question for you, but I do hope I've given you enough information to help you make the decision for yourself or a loved one. This is your process and your decision; I'm not telling you what to do, but I am letting you know about your options and sharing my perspective. I'm not your doctor, therapist, lawyer or guru. I hope to answer whatever questions you may have, but you have to find your own answers.

Where we are going with cannabis and how it can be tailored in ever-finer ways is complex. The plant's total cannabinoid profile and your individual physiology can work together in sophisticated and incredibly effective ways. The number of ways and forms to consume, along with all the strains available, gives us a toolkit packed with countless possibilities.

If you do choose to move forward, I hope I've given you the guidance and direction to do so with confidence. You have plenty of options to consume safely, discreetly and comfortably. You know to take it low and slow, especially with the edibles. You know to pay attention to cannabinoid profiles and THC/CBD ratios. You're aware that it may take some experimentation to find your sweet spot. You're prepared for some variability but trust your experience will never get too bad (and now you have the tools to bring you down if it does…CBD, remember?) You know it can be used with other medications, but you also know they might need to be adjusted. You can do it!

Before You Go

I'll wrap it up now—but will recap our conversation and impart these final words of wisdom:

Take control: Do your homework and know what you want from your experience (and what you don't want). Blind choices are bad choices.

Take your time: Don't feel rushed or pressured. Ask questions. Acknowledge your canna-newb status and ask for help or clarification. We're chill. It's all good!

Go low and slow: Don't set yourself up for a bad experience. Be patient, follow the process. Don't go overboard. Common sense, use it.

Respect the plant*:* Do consume consciously and with intention and appreciation. It may be referred to as weed, but cannabis is complex and multi-dimensional. Remember, she's a mother, too.

Be reasonable: Don't expect miracles. Anything is possible, but nothing fixes everything. There are no guarantees. Be open, but don't be a fool. Beware the snake oil and sales pitches. Be optimistic, but be real.

Behave responsibly: Don't flake out and put yourself or others at risk. Safety first, always. Be prepared. Know the laws and regulations, and know your rights. Know your limits. Break the stigma, don't reinforce it.

Respect yourself and others*:* Do take care of yourself. Use marijuana for your highest and best interest. Don't use it as a coping tool or to check out of life or relationships. Be aware of the relationship you have with weed. Be aware of the people around you. We've got to love one another right now.

You do you*:* Don't feel shame or embarrassment. If you choose to consume cannabis, for whatever reasons, own it. If it's legally available and you're an adult, then there's nothing wrong with it. You're a grown-up. You don't need permission. You get to choose what's right for you.

No matter what, it will all be okay: Don't be afraid. You can't die or overdose (and if you live by the low-and-slow credo, you won't over dose.) You won't get addicted. Your mind will be enhanced, not altered. Chances are, your fears are completely unfounded. Come on in, the water is fine.

I've done my best to make this very complex and nuanced topic understandable, digestible and somewhat actionable. You're getting a wealth of information in the book, but I'm also giving you some Cliff's Notes, so to speak. I hope I've given you enough knowledge and confidence to take whatever next steps make sense for you or a loved one. And that might just be none. But you'll do it with choice and not because of false beliefs and unfounded fears.

I encourage you to keep asking questions, for yourself and your family. Cannabis is changing the paradigm. There's more information and knowledge available every day. More products and options on the market to consider. We are all learning as we go, there is no roadmap to follow. This is a conversation, not a monologue.

I'll be following up this book with a website (wakinguptoweed.com) to help answer more questions, provide further information and resources, share updates and build a community where people like you can find the tools and support to be a confident, conscientious cannabis consumer. Come ask questions and share your stories (from inside or out of the canna closet.) We're all in this together—the more we all know and the more we all share with each other, the more we can help not just the people we care about the most, but the people like you who are seeking answers to their questions about cannabis.

Let's keep the conversation going, I can't wait to hear about your experience!

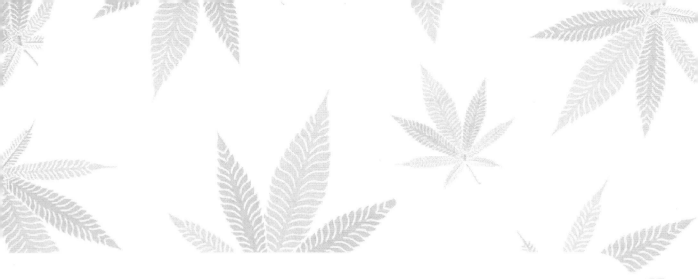

CLOSING QUESTION:

So when all is said and done, is weed for me? Or perhaps, someone I love?

I cannot answer the question of whether cannabis is for you or someone you love. It's possible. It's helping a lot of people in a lot of ways. From hardcore medical application to simple life enhancement, weed wears a lot of hats. Takes on a lot of forms and plays a lot of roles. It has minimal downside, no actual physical risk and while the evidence is still coming, seems to offer a lot of potential to deliver quantifiable value, regardless of how that value is quantified or measured. If it's an option for you or a loved one, I highly recommend you consider it. And if you do move forward in some way, do it conscientiously and with the knowledge I've shared here, and you can do it with confidence.

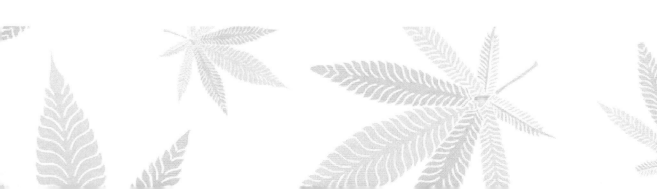

RESOURCES & FURTHER READING

Remember folks, knowledge is power. And, when it comes to weed, there is always something new to know. I encourage you to dig deeper into questions you have and topics that spark your interest, and to make conscious choices about cannabis consumption. The overblown risks of death and destruction are myths, but that doesn't mean it's risk free. Do your homework and continue to get educated. Make informed decisions.

And if the door to your canna closet is open, step out into the light. Break the stigma. Get involved. Help others wake up and see what might be possible with cannabis.

Here are a few resources to get you started, see where the path takes you!

Organizations

NORML
http://norml.org/
202.483.5500

Students for Sensible Drug Policy (SSDP)
https://ssdp.org/
202.393.5280

Marijuana Policy Project (MPP)
www.mpp.org
202.462.5747

Drug Policy Alliance (DPA)
www.drugpolicy.org
212.613.8020

Law Enforcement Against Prohibition (LEAP)
www.leap.cc
781.393.6985

Americans for Safe Access
www.safeaccessnow.org
202.857.4272

Multidisciplinary Association for Psychedelic Studies (MAPS)
http://www.maps.org/
831.429.MDMA (6362)

IMPACT Network
https://www.impactcannabis.org/

Online Resources

Marijuana Laws by State
http://norml.org/laws

Marijuana Research
http://norml.org/library

CBD Research
https://www.projectcbd.org/

Medical Cannabis
https://www.medicaljane.com/

News & Information
www.thecannabist.co/
https://www.leafly.com/

Books

Cannabis for Chronic Pain:
A Proven Prescription for Using Marijuana to
Relieve Your Pain and Heal Your Life
by Dr. Rav Ivker

The Cannabis Manifesto:
A New Paradigm for Wellness
by Steve DeAngelo

Vitamin Wed: A 4-Step Plan to Preventing and Reversing
Endocannabinoid Deficiency
by Dr. Michele Ross, Ph.D.

The Cannabis Kitchen Cookbook:
Feel-Good Food for Home Cooks
by Robyn Griggs Lawrence

Cannabis and Spirituality:
An Explorer's Guide to an Ancient Plant Spirit Ally
by Stephen Gray

Marijuana Grower's Handbook:
Your Complete Guide for Medical and
Personal Marijuana Cultivation
by Ed Rosenthal

acknowledgments

THANK
YOU

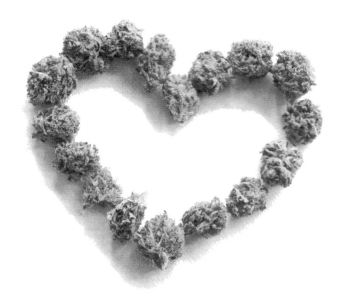

I've jokingly referred to this book as my "weed baby" as I've carried it from concept through gestation. It was an unplanned pregnancy, so to speak; an immaculate "cannaception" that perhaps unironically, took 9 months from the spark of an idea to its birth. I'm deeply grateful to the people surrounding and supporting me throughout its gestation, I may be the equivalent of a single mother, but I'm far from alone.

This book would never have happened without the inspiration and insight of my dear friend, Jill Davis. You showed me what's possible and you continue to light the way for me, and for so many other aspiring writers and speakers. You have more impact than you can possibly imagine—for such a little fairy, your pixie dust packs some punch. You are this weed baby's godmother; she's lucky to have your joy and wisdom to guide her. (And to Jill Buckingham, thank you for both the name and the sparks of hope that keep me going in the darkest times.)

This weed baby would never have made it into the world without James Woosley of Free Agent Press, who helps independent authors like myself birth their own books. I appreciate your guidance, patience and fortitude as we've brought this book to bear—you've kept your calm and kept me together through this roller coaster ride, no easy task. I hope if you've been compelled to try consumption along the way, it's because of the content of the book and not the process behind creating it!

I'm also blessed to have had support from some amazingly talented creative and publishing professionals, who each sprinkled their fairy dust in their own way along the way. Heartfelt thanks and appreciation to Raelina Krikston for your efforts and ideas; I look forward to the day when we can do it right. Deep gratitude as well to Mike Romane and Jamie Johnston; you are design rock stars and I appreciate you both. Michael Heckler took my head shots and only the sun made me cringe; thank you for battling the cold to help capture my shine. Jennifer Harshman made sure I had my i's dotted and t's crossed, and Michelle Vandepas made sure I had myself positioned for success. And Jaime Mintun gave me more resources, support and strength than I could have possibly asked; I can't wait to see what we manifest.

The cannabis community has shown me what's possible when good people come together to advance a cause and build meaningful businesses. I admire your passion, hustle and shared desire to connect people to this plant. Keep it going, you all are forging the path. To Holly Alberti-Evans I send my gratitude, love and, of course, my chi; thank you for being you. You're a warrior and I appreciate all you do to help others rise higher every day. And to Charles Jones, thank you for seeing what's possible and opening the door for me and so many others. The world needs more awake CEOs and I'm thrilled you are in the vanguard.

Any woman would be lucky to have the support of the friends and family that surrounds this weed baby and me. I would never have started on this path without the foundation laid by Todd, who taught me to love the plant and myself. I could never have found my way without the shining beacon of light coming from Kim, who has shown me, and so many others, the power and potential of love and healing. Thank you and the rest of the Tribe for being my biggest cheerleaders and being with me through every step of the journey. I couldn't have done it without you. And I really couldn't have done this, or anything for that matter, without the lifelong support, guidance and love of my folks, James and Susan. You have provided every opportunity for me and are a testament to good parenting. There are no words for my love and gratitude.

This weed baby is going to come into the world with so much love and support, thank you all for helping make it a world worth coming into. With love and appreciation – S.

STEPHANIE BYER

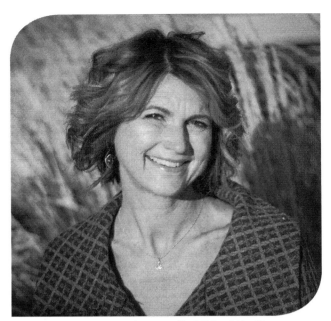

photo credit: Michael Heckler

Stephanie Byer is a writer, communicator, consultant, speaker, coach, strategist, cancer survivor and cannavangelist. She is a former communications and strategy executive who found a 'higher purpose' in cannabis, with a mission to help people see what's possible with weed. She has woken up to its benefits, using marijuana to overcome opioid dependence and manage chronic pain, as an alternative to alcohol and to ease depression and anxiety. Stephanie wrote *Waking Up to Weed* to help people see what's possible and feel more comfortable considering cannabis for themselves or a loved one.

Before turned she started educating and talking to people about cannabis, Stephanie helped them navigate choices and complex information so they could make better financial and healthcare decisions. She spent 25 years working with corporations and entrepreneurs to create more meaningful communications and experiences for people. Stephanie graduated from the University of Michigan and holds an MBA from DePaul University.

She has been, and continues to be, dedicated to elevating people's perception of and their experience with cannabis—not just with the plant itself, but with the people and brands bringing this market into the mainstream. She lives and enjoys the high life in Denver, CO with her rescue dog Diesel (named after her favorite strain of weed, Sour Diesel!)

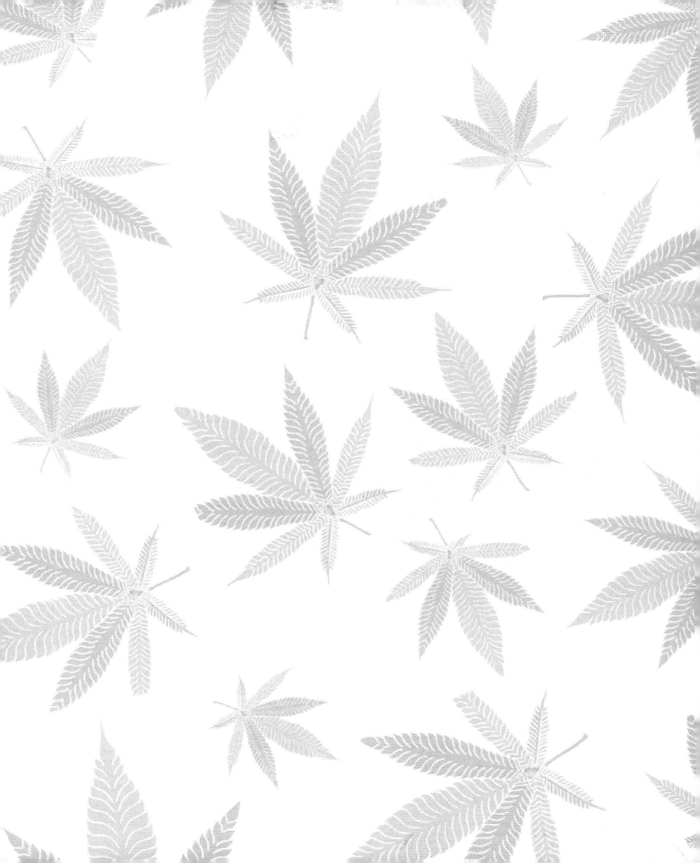

Learn More at

WakingUpToWeed.com

Made in the USA
San Bernardino, CA
22 February 2018